LISA RILEY'S
Honesty
DIET

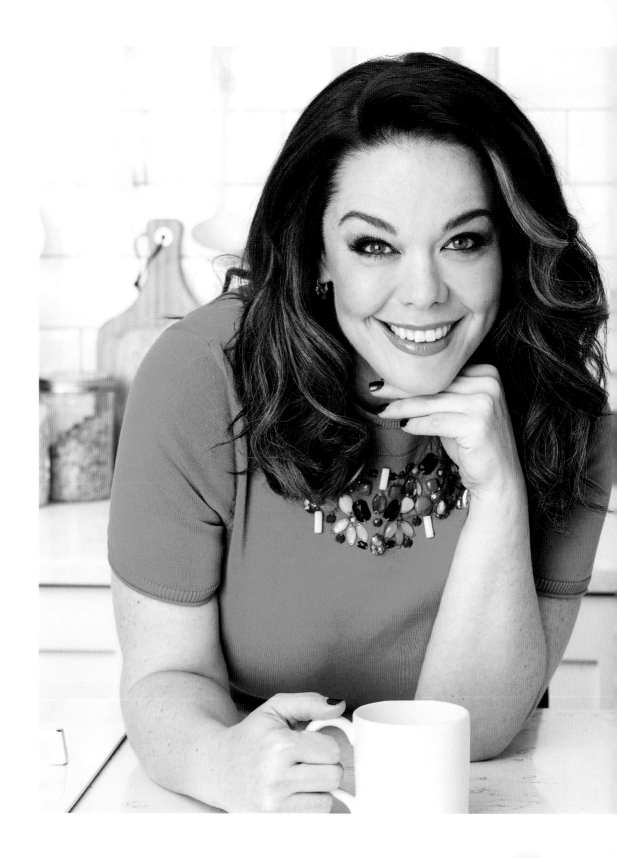

LISA RILEY'S Honesty DIET

Change your life in just 8 days

MICHAEL JOSEPH
an imprint of
PENGUIN BOOKS

MICHAEL JOSEPH
UK | USA | Canada | Ireland | Australia
India | New Zealand | South Africa

Michael Joseph is part of the Penguin Random House
group of companies whose addresses can be found at
global.penguinrandomhouse.com

Penguin
Random House
UK

First published 2017
001

Edited by Jordan Paramor

Design and layout by HART STUDIO

Hair and make-up by Tracey Jones

Food styling and recipe development by Kat Mead

Prop styling by Jemima Hetherington

Colour reproduction by Altaimage Ltd
Printed in Germany by Mohn Media

A CIP catalogue record for this book is available
from the British Library

ISBN: 978–0–718–18887–0

www.greenpenguin.co.uk

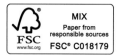

Penguin Random House is committed to a
sustainable future for our business, our readers
and our planet. This book is made from Forest
Stewardship Council® certified paper.

This book is for Al (Bubby): my love, my best friend, my rock and my shield. You came to me from an angel in the sky, and all this happened because you made me fly.

For Dad, Liam, Nat, Jakey and Joshua: never stop looking for the smile in the moon.

And for my beloved mum, Cath Riley, my ever-present angel. Her legacy lives on for ever in me.

CONTENTS

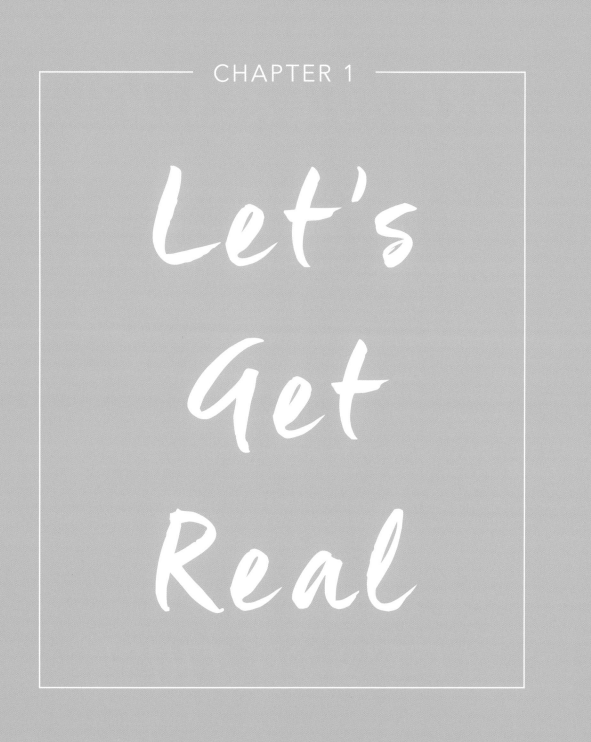

CHAPTER 1

Let's Get Real

ARE YOU READY?!

Are you ready to lose weight?

Are you ready to get honest?

Are you ready to hear things you may not like?

Are you ready to feel incredible?

Are you ready to discover the real you?

Are you ready to work hard?

Are you ready to break through the pain barrier?

Are you ready to see your body transform?

If you answered yes to all of these questions, your life is about to change beyond recognition.

I'm telling you now that you can and will lose weight.

LET'S DO THIS!

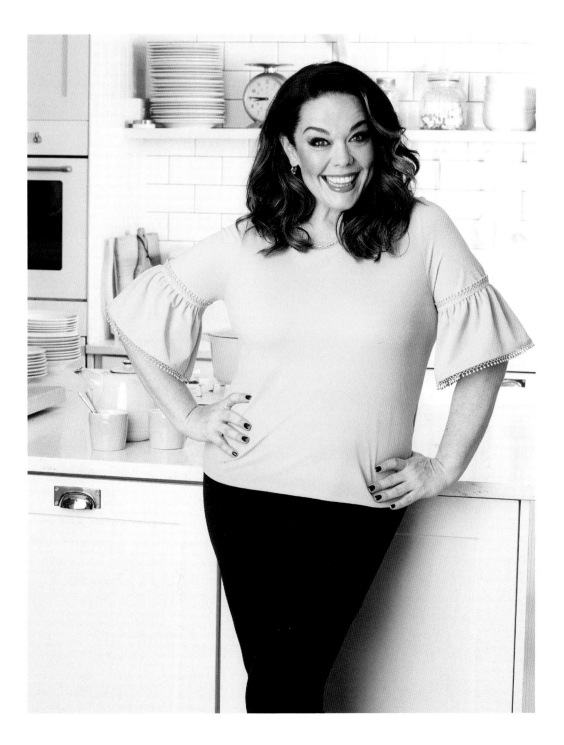

WELCOME

Welcome to what I hope will be a life-changing book for you. My own life has changed beyond belief over the past couple of years, and now I want to share everything I've learned on my weight-loss journey.

I've called this book my Honesty Diet because that's exactly what it is. You're going to be honest with yourself; other people are going to be honest with you; and you're going to be honest about every single thing you put in your mouth.

You're not going to get to the middle of this book and find a magic weight-loss pill hidden within the pages. The reason? It doesn't exist.

If you're serious about losing weight, the only way it's going to happen is if you:
- eat healthier meals
- choose smaller portions
- move around more

This book is all about honesty, so I'm going to start off by sharing a pretty hard truth with you:

IF YOU'RE OVERWEIGHT, YOU'RE EATING TOO MUCH!

Are you ready for some more tough love?

IF YOU'RE OVERWEIGHT, YOU'RE ALSO PROBABLY NOT MOVING AROUND ENOUGH

The diet industry doesn't want you to know that weight loss is as simple as eating less and moving more. They want you to keep buying their low-fat, additive-laden products, and losing weight/putting it back on again at expensive slimming clubs. Why would they give you a long-term, common sense, sustainable plan when instead they can keep making more money from you, over and over and over?

ENOUGH NOW!

I'm not about to give you false promises or tell you that you can still eat what you want and lose weight, because you can't. I'm not one of those people who's going to say you can eat chocolate and ice cream and still drop pounds, because that's simply not true.

If you're looking for a super-quick fix or for someone else to do the work for you, then this isn't the diet for you. And in the spirit of honesty I want to say upfront that there are some bits you may find tough. Nothing worth having was ever easy!

But the incredible news? It really does bloody work.

Just look at me. This plan will be hard at times but it will change your body.

This isn't one of those diets to do for a couple of months and then get complacent about. If you want to feel amazing for the rest of your life you have to be mindful and honest about what you're eating at all times.

Dieting will always be a way of life for me now. People notice all the time that I'm 'careful', but that's because I have to be. Being really focused on what I eat is what gets results and keeps me where I want to be.

The proof is in the pudding. (Or, in this case, in not having the pudding!) I am walking, talking, smiling evidence that with the right guidance, determination and self-belief (and a healthy dose of willpower) you can be the size you've always wanted to be.

Back when I was delving into my wardrobe and pulling out size 28 clothes, I never dreamed I'd be able to walk into a shop and pick up a size 12 knowing it would fit me. But now that's my reality every time I buy new clothes. And my God, I love it! I cannot describe the buzz I get when I wear something from a shop I used to stare wistfully into as I made my way to the plus size stores.

I cried my eyes out when I first put on a size 12 T-shirt. It was the best feeling ever. A friend of mine said to me that I was smiling so much at that moment I was glowing. I want each and every one of you to experience that very same feeling.

Here's another thing you may not want to hear: I'm not the slimming fairy and I don't have a magic wand. Only you can put in the work and drop dress sizes.

It's also not enough just to read this book. You have to take action!

So throw those crisps in the bin, dust off your trainers, and prepare for the fabulous new you!

YOUR NEW BEST FRIEND

Well, actually, you're going to have two.

The first one is me. By the time you've finished reading this book, hopefully you'll hear my voice in your head like a concerned friend every time you want to sneak to the corner shop and stock up on Doritos.

I want you to know that I'm rooting for you every step of the way. And I'm not just here in book form. You can follow me on Facebook, Twitter and Instagram, and I'll try to reply to messages whenever I can. You can also interact online with other people who are working to lose weight, and I can tell you from experience that you'll get tons of support. Use #honestydiet to find other people on a similar path to you.

Your second best friend is going to be your Honesty Diary (see pages 18–19). From now on, you're going to write down every little thing you eat so it's in front of you in black and white – or whatever colour ink you like best!

Buy yourself a brand-new notebook or diary so you can start afresh. It doesn't have to be expensive, but it's going to be with you for a long time so make sure you love it.

From now on, you are your own:
- diet coach
- personal trainer
- therapist (sometimes!)

And, even better, you come for free!

Any time you feel up or down, make a note of it. Record what you're feeling and anything specific that happened to make you feel that way.

You may laugh, it's entirely possible you'll cry, and you'll probably be pretty amazed about how much denial you've been in. That's all brilliant. I shed a fair few tears in those early days, I can tell you. Then, later on down the line, they turned to tears of joy.

There's a good chance you'll be shocked about what you've been doing to yourself all these years. Not just about what you've been consuming, but the negative messages you've been literally 'feeding' yourself, and how much of a hard time you've been giving yourself for 'failing' at dieting.

You haven't failed at dieting. You just weren't coming at it from the right angle.

I can't stress enough how much of a game changer it was for me when I acknowledged what I was eating on a daily basis. Once I was realistic about the fact *I* was the one who had made – and was keeping – myself fat, I was able to start making real, substantial changes.

It's so important to write things down and face them. Over the years, I'd told so many lies to myself about losing weight, I'd completely deafened myself with them. I constantly told myself, 'I can't,' and 'I won't.' I'd got used to being different from other people and labelling myself the 'fat, funny one'. Until I recognized that the only person I was lying to about the mess I'd got myself into was me, I couldn't move on.

The more emotions that you express and are honest about, the better you'll feel, and the more you can begin to understand what's been going on beneath the surface.

People only see the excess pounds, but weight problems run so much deeper than that. This is why I want to help you find out your triggers and pitfalls, so that you can confront them.

I have confidence in you!

I know you're going to do such a great job with this that, by the end of the process, *you'll* want the best for you, just like I do. You won't want to let yourself down.

These days, I live and breathe honesty. I've always been honest with other people, but now I'm honest with myself too. I don't lie to myself ever. And it's time for you to do the same. Want to know a secret?

THE MORE HONEST WITH YOURSELF YOU ARE, THE BIGGER THE CHANGE YOU'LL SEE!

GET TO KNOW YOUR
EATING HABITS

To get the ball rolling I'd like you to fill in this questionnaire. It will help you to start thinking about the way you eat, and why.

You can either write your answers directly in the book, or copy the questions down into your Honesty Diary and answer them in there.

You can reread your answers and add to them at any point. It might be interesting to see how your responses change over time. They will be really important in the coming months, so write as much as you want to. There is no limit.

Remember, the answers are just for you, and no one else has to read them. So be one hundred per cent – wait for it – HONEST!

Now take some time to read through your answers. When you get to the last six, give yourself time to really absorb and process them.

Feel how you're going to feel wearing that outfit. Imagine yourself smiling when you look in the mirror at your gorgeous new figure. And tell yourself how much you deserve to feel fabulous.

Draw a picture of yourself in your head – or in your notebook, if you fancy getting a bit arty.

Hold on to that image.

Make it come alive.

THAT'S YOUR FUTURE, RIGHT THERE!

When did your weight
problems start?

What do you think triggered them?

Was there one thing that changed
your eating habits?

Did you get comments about your
weight when you were growing up?

What is the worst thing anyone's
ever said to you about your weight?

How did you react/deal with it?

Looking back, was there a better
way you could have dealt with it?

On a scale of 1–10, how much is your
weight bothering you right now?

What bothers you the most about
your weight?

What do you wish you could wear
that you can't at the moment?

What would be your dream outfit?

If you were slimmer, what would you do that you don't do now?

Which foods are your biggest downfalls?

Do you know when to stop eating?

Do you think you eat the right portion sizes?

Are you a big snacker?

Do you reward yourself with food?

Would you say you're in denial about how much you really eat?

Are the people around you helpful when it comes to your eating patterns?

Do you comfort eat when you're low?

What are your triggers?

Is there anything you could do to change or resist your triggers?
(This is a tough one, but think about it.)

What is the kindest thing you could do for yourself right now?

Why do you deserve to lose weight?

Is there a reason you don't deserve to lose weight? (Challenge anything you write down after this question. Is it really true? My guess is probably not. Imagine a friend said to you what you've just said to yourself. How would you feel? What would you say in response?)

How will you feel once you reach your goal weight?

How will you celebrate?

How did you react/deal with it?

In what ways do you think it will be different doing everyday things?

How are you going to feel when you're wearing that dream outfit?

What will you dare to do that you've always been too scared to do?

How big is the smile on your face going to be when you wake up feeling incredible every morning?

THE HONESTY DIARY

This is how I laid out my own Honesty Diary. Every day I wrote down:

- what time I ate
- what I ate
- why I ate it
- how it made me feel

Each night, when I went to bed, I wrote a brief summary of my day, and I went to sleep holding the image of the all-new future me in my head.

Copy the grid opposite into your Honesty Diary or simply photocopy it lots of times. Alternatively. you could write it on to a chalkboard or whiteboard, or even your kids' easel, if you've got one.

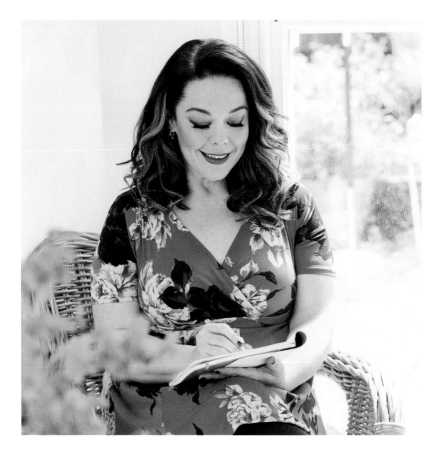

DATE	TIME	WHAT?	WHY?	HOW DID I FEEL?
BREAKFAST				
LUNCH				
DINNER				
SNACKS				
SUMMARY OF THE DAY				

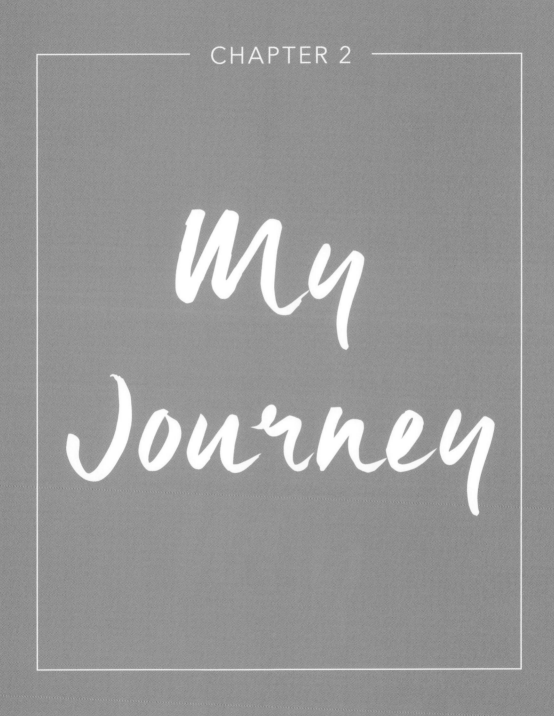

CHAPTER 2

My Journey

MY JOURNEY

People often ask if I've always been a 'big girl'. The truth is I've always had a tendency to be a bit overweight, but nothing like the weight I ended up reaching.

I was a plump child but I wasn't fat. Fridays used to be treat night, when I'd go round to my grandparents' house and watch *Dynasty*. My granddad would pop to the corner kiosk and get me two litres of Tizer, a bag of Quavers and a Twix or a Caramac bar. Quite often he'd buy both and I'd happily eat them, so it's fair to say that I always liked my treats.

By the time I hit puberty, and got to around thirteen or fourteen, I was definitely bigger than all the girls in my class. I was also quite short, which made me look dumpy. It wasn't just that I was unlucky with my weight. I ate all the wrong things, and way too much of them. Like most kids, I liked crisps, sweets and fizzy drinks, but, while most kids grow out of them or learn about moderation, I carried on enjoying them to excess.

People were always telling me the extra pounds were just puppy fat and would disappear as I grew up. But instead I grew outwards. I remember all my friends wearing these tracksuits that were fashionable when we were in our teens, but I was too big to fit into one. I was gutted but I told myself things wouldn't be like that forever.

It wasn't like I was lazy. I actually did quite a lot of exercise growing up because I went to drama school from the age of nine, and there we danced a lot. But the bottom line was I ate too much. And whenever I ate, I consumed junk food. Lots of it.

When I was fourteen my mum took me to a dietician because she was worried my weight was getting a bit out of control. Dieticians are experts in nutrition. They advise people who have certain health conditions or who are over- or underweight, so my mum was hopeful they could steer me down a healthier path and help me to lose weight.

It was not a good experience. The dietician patronized the hell out of me and told me I had to live on a high-fibre diet for the rest of my life. She told me to stick to foods like baked potatoes, brown bread and beans – which I've since learned is terrible advice. Of course there are many great dieticians out there, and nutritional science has moved on since I was a kid, but I guess I saw the wrong person back then and was quite unlucky with the advice I was given.

I told myself being overweight was in my genes. I couldn't blame my mum, though, because she was never a big lady. She was only a size 10 on her wedding day. But my dad is a larger chap, so I assumed I must have taken after him, and I used it as an excuse whenever I put on more weight.

I was a pretty big girl by the time I got my role in *Emmerdale*, aged eighteen, and that was really the beginning of me becoming properly obese. My character, Mandy, was a tomboy 'rugger bugger' type so it suited her to be big, and I got larger as time went on. I partly blame the studio catering and the snack trolley. But, let's face it, no one was force-feeding me.

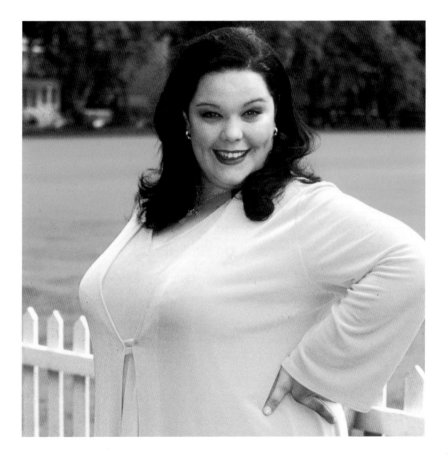

When I landed a role on the ITV drama series *Fat Friends* it didn't even cross my mind that it was because I was so heavy. It was just an amazing show to be a part of, and they'd cast me because they knew I would do a great job on it. The fact I was fat was by the by.

I'm very lucky that, in spite of my size, I've always been really confident – and probably in denial about how big I was – so it didn't bother me hugely. If it ever did, I'd switch on what I call the 'BB' – the bravado button – and pretend not to care. That was my trick when I was feeling a bit self-conscious. I'd laugh a bit louder, and then eat another biscuit.

I think if my career had dipped and I'd thought it was down to my weight, I probably would have done something about it. But it didn't, and I was working constantly. Of course I always got cast in fat roles, but I learned to style it out. I was 'the fat, funny one' from the telly. But I guess at some point it stopped being funny for me. Eventually I ran out of punchlines to justify how big I was.

I knew there were some roles I'd simply never get, such as sexy seductress parts. I wholeheartedly accepted that was just the way it was, and probably always would be. I won't lie; there were some roles I would have *loved* but knew I would never land. There were so many great police dramas being made in Manchester, and I was desperate to play a detective or a forensic investigator. I love dark, gritty dramas. But I didn't ever get called for auditions.

It's crazy how things change, because now I'm slim I'm already getting roles I know I would never have been considered for before. It feels incredible. These days I'm being chosen and judged for my acting ability, and not just because I've got a particular body shape. A friend of mine recently told me that she loves the fact I no longer play only downtrodden characters. Now I can play feisty, happy women too!

There have been some very unkind things written about me and my size in the press over the years, but I reasoned that I'd put myself in the spotlight and that was the pay-off. I learned to block things out, but one time I found really tough was when I was about twenty-seven and some paparazzi pictures were taken of me on the beach while I was on holiday. It was just bad luck that a journalist happened to be staying in the same hotel as me, and they tipped off a photographer. The next thing I knew, my body was splashed across the pages of a tabloid in a swimsuit.

One of the Sunday newspapers ran the photos along with the headline 'Emmerwhale'. Yes, I looked massive and the pictures were revolting, but it was still very unkind. The worst thing for me was that the piece was written by a female reporter. For some reason it hurt a lot more that a woman had taken it upon herself to be so vitriolic about my figure. Aren't we girls supposed to stick together? Personally, I think so.

I wasn't embarrassed when I saw the photos; I was disgusted. I was made to feel like I'd done something terribly wrong simply because I was big. I hadn't murdered anyone. But apparently – because I was obese – I may as well have done. A girl recently messaged me online saying that she's made to feel like a modern-day leper because she's fat, and I totally identify with that.

I was mortified that my friends and family saw those photos, and I didn't want them to be upset on my behalf. I honestly think, if I wasn't as confident as I am, that single article could have destroyed me and killed my career. Even though I refused to let it do so, it did take me a while to get my 'oomph' back afterwards.

I was one of a group of famous women – along with the likes of Dawn French, Caroline Quentin and Jo Brand – who were put in what I call 'the fat cauldron'. The press were always watching to see if we'd lost or put on weight, and it felt like a lot of pressure. Looking back, it's probably one of the things that made me think 'sod it' as I munched my way through yet another Chinese takeaway.

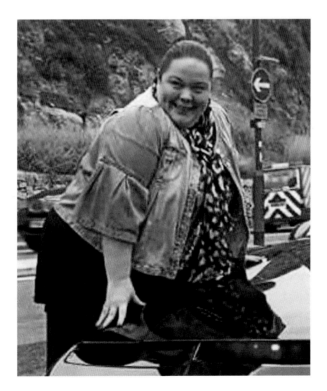

STRICTLY SLIMMING?

As many of you will know, I took part in the fabulous *Strictly Come Dancing* in 2012. It was an unbelievable experience and, if I could, I'd go back and do it all again tomorrow. A lot of people assume that's where my weight-loss journey must have started. But, while it did help me to fall back in love with exercise, in some ways my eating habits became worse than ever.

When I was first offered a part in the show I had to think really long and hard about it. My mum had passed away in my arms just weeks before, so I wasn't in a great place emotionally. I was also worried that people would judge me.

And what about the clothes? Most of the women wore the equivalent of sparkling bathing suits. What were they going to do with me? Decorate a garden umbrella with sequins and cut out holes for my arms?

I didn't want to be the 'different' one who couldn't wear pretty outfits. Every fat person who had been on *Strictly* before had been the token comedy one. Did I want to be that person? I knew I could dance, but would anyone take me seriously when I was the size I was?

Was I chosen for *Strictly* because I was a size 28? Maybe. Did I care? Not in the end.

The producers knew I could move and that people would be shocked when they saw me on the dance floor. They knew it would have an impact. I had to believe in that too, and be brave enough to take the chance.

Although I wasn't feeling my best when I signed up for the series, when I look back now I can see it was the most positive thing I could have done at that unhappy time in my life. It gave me a real focus. I wanted to learn everything and soak it all up. I didn't ever want to stop rehearsing. My wonderful partner, Robin Windsor, used to say, 'We're done for the day,' and I'd be like, 'No, I want more!' That was after six hours of dancing, too.

The first night I danced in front of the public was amazing because I went out there ready to stick two fingers up to anyone who thought I wouldn't be able to move well. A newspaper review the next day said, 'Lisa Riley is very light on her feet.' They may as well have added #forafatbird.

Robin and I found ways around things. For instance, because I was too heavy for him to lift, I ended up lifting *him*. I'm proud to say that, to this day, I'm the only woman on the show ever to lift up a male partner. Sometimes you've got to break the rules!

I hadn't considered that weight loss might be a side effect of doing the show because I'd accepted that I was always going to be fat. But a couple of weeks into the show an amazing thing happened.

All the dancers had a mannequin that was set to our exact measurements, so the costumiers could make sure outfits fitted us perfectly, and all of a sudden they had to make mine smaller. I was naturally losing weight – thanks to all the non-stop exercise I was doing. I was becoming fitter and slimmer doing something I enjoyed, which gave me a real buzz.

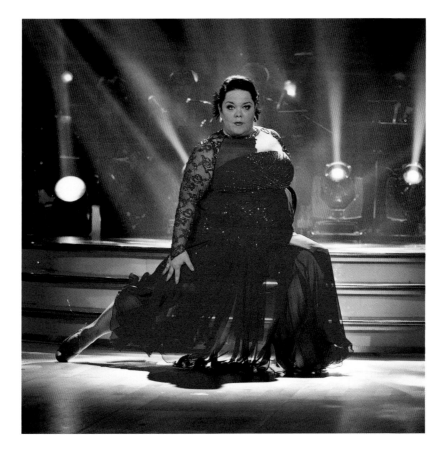

But, although all the exercise was giving my metabolism a kick-start, the problem was that I was still very much in my 'old Lisa' mindset, with all my bad food habits. I stupidly told myself that I could eat *more* because I was doing so much cardio, and that's exactly what I did.

Every Tuesday, on the way to the rehearsal studio, Robin and I used to buy all the new gossip magazines and a ton of chocolate and crisps. Then we'd lie on the floor of the rehearsal studio and wolf down the lot. I used the fact I was exercising a lot as an excuse to eat more crap. So, instead of losing more weight over the coming weeks, it kind of evened back out.

I went on the *Strictly* tour shortly after the series finished, which was another killer because the tour bus was constantly stocked up with sweets, crisps, cheese sandwiches and wine. I'd have a full English in our hotel each morning, and then take a couple of breakfast muffins for the journey.

We'd stop at a service station a couple of hours later and I'd grab some tubes of Pringles and a trifle. Not an individual one, mind. One of those that said 'family' on the top.

Every night my dressing room was full of Millie's Cookies and bars of chocolate. It was so bad that Artem, one of the professional dancers, walked into my dressing room one night and joked I had so many Twix bars I could have built my own railway line with them as the sleepers. And that's not to mention all the post-show red wine I enjoyed.

The dancers ate a lot, but that's because they had to. They dance so much they actually need the extra calories to keep their weight up. I wasn't doing six hours of rehearsals a day any more, but I was still eating as if I was.

After the *Strictly* tour finished, Craig Revel Horwood very kindly wrote me my own musical, called *Strictly Confidential*. So I was soon back on the road, and the calorie binge carried on.

I was dancing for an hour and a half a night, and then telling myself because I'd exercised it was fine to go back to the hotel and polish off cheese and onion toasties with crisps and wine at midnight. Not surprisingly, the weight piled on. And the pounds brought friends with them.

Although *Strictly* didn't prove to be the start of my weight-loss journey, it did help to change my attitude. It showed me that I was capable of losing weight if I put my mind to it. But I'd have to put in the work and change my eating habits. It would still be a little while before I was ready to tackle this, though.

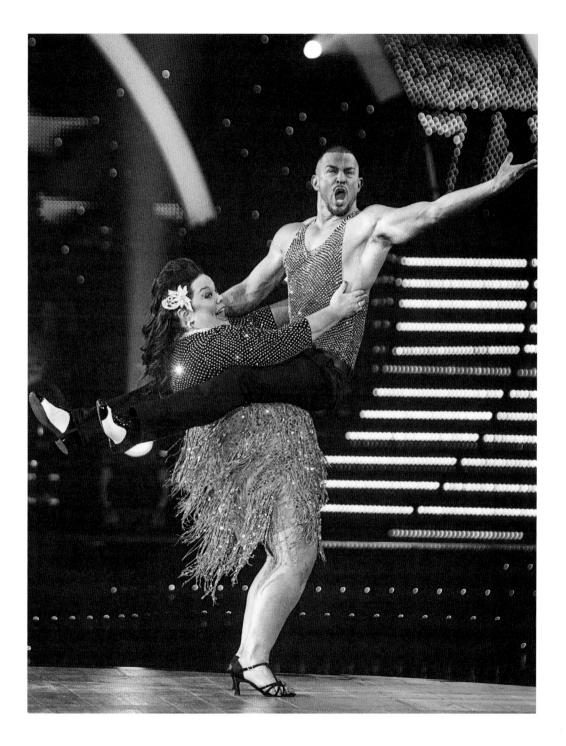

MY MAIN WEIGHT DOWNFALLS

You may just recognize some of these!

I WAS THE QUEEN OF CARBS

I always, *always* had a Warburtons white loaf in the bread bin. I'd eat it toasted, with so much butter it would swim around on top. It was like a buttery pond. Insects could have swum in it.

When the 4 p.m. snack trolley came round when I was on set filming, I'd wolf down huge prawn sandwiches with tons of butter, as well as doughnuts and cakes. This was after I'd eaten a big lunch.

I also lived on every kind of potatoes. Baked potatoes, chips, mash – you name it. Crisps will always be one of my weaknesses, and that will probably never go away. If you were to wave a bag of Kettle Chips around in front of me, I'd wilt. I used to be able to polish off a tube of Pringles in minutes, and then go back for more. Whenever I packed to go away somewhere, I'd throw a couple of bags of crisps in my suitcase, and often another one in my handbag – just in case I got peckish.

I'd never been a confident cook (I'm still no Delia, but I do try), so when my family came round for dinner I always made the same thing: a meat lasagne and a Quorn lasagne with baked potatoes. Double carbs! And then I'd serve bread on the side! Whenever we went to my brother's, he made mac 'n' cheese with garlic bread, and I'd eat it like I was never going to eat again.

I ADORED SUGAR

I was always picking at sweets. I'd have a few bags on the go, and I was constantly dipping in and out. Even now, I have to try really hard to stop myself if people offer me an open bag.

I also had a massive weakness for coffee and walnut cake. If someone mentions it, I still start to salivate. I'm only human! It's such a favourite that I've included a healthier version of it in my recipe section (see page 250). It's only for end-of-plan rewards, mind you!

I LOVED EATING OUT

I love Italian food, and I'd always have pasta and garlic bread. I never ate less than three courses, plus sides, and a chocolate dessert and a milky coffee to finish. (When did it become law that you must eat three courses when you go out?) Then I'd often stop on the way home and get some Pringles and chocolate to eat while watching TV.

I WAS CONSTANTLY PUSHING MY 'F*** IT' BUTTON

I was so good at saying to myself, 'I shouldn't have that, but f*** it!'

If I had a sandwich, I had a giant one. If I had a slice of cake, I'd quickly polish off the rest of it.

Every time that little voice in my head said, 'Are you sure you should be doing this?' I'd push that button, and I'd push it hard.

WHY DIDN'T ANYONE SAY ANYTHING?

The weird thing is, I was never self-conscious about how much I ate, and I'd happily munch away in front of people. I thought it was normal. I didn't imagine that people were looking at me and thinking, 'Wow, she's greedy!'

Crazily, no one ever said anything to me about how much I ate, either. How on earth not? They must have noticed.

One time, I went to a new burger restaurant that had opened in Manchester. I had a starter, a veggie burger, triple-cooked chips, a side of onion rings, a chocolate brownie and wine. I talked about it with such affection for weeks afterwards. What must people have thought?

My friends used to call me an 'extremist'. I translated that into being 'the giddy one' and 'the one who drinks a lot of wine'. But did they really mean I was extreme with food?

Friends have since told me that they were worried about me being so big. But no one said a word at the time. I do wish they'd said something to me back then, but I appreciate how difficult it is.

I've asked my friends why they never broached the subject of my weight. They've all said they were too frightened, which I completely understand. They were too scared of what my reaction would be. They also thought I was genuinely happy and that I was just 'being me'. The fact that everyone was terrified to tell it like it was is the reason I came up with the idea of having an Honesty Buddy.

THE POWER OF THE HONESTY BUDDY

The Honesty Buddy can be quite a daunting concept, but it's really important – so stick with me!

What I want you to do is to choose a family member, or a friend you love and trust, and ask them to be completely honest with you at all times while you're following this plan. They're allowed to tell you off if you're cheating, point out whenever you look like you're about to fall off the wagon, and stop you reaching for that packet of Chelsea buns. If they're too scared to say anything to your face (though I recommend you pick someone brave), give them permission to text or email you. Ask them for tough love. But you have to agree to forgive them if they pull you up on things.

My Honesty Buddy was my partner, Al. I couldn't have embarked on my journey without his help. I was so grateful to have someone in my life who was with me all the way. He helped me stay on track when things became really challenging. He was amazingly supportive, but also tough when I needed him to be.

Remember that your nearest and dearest want to be helpful, not hurtful, and you'll thank them for it down the line. An honest friend can make all the difference. Having a support network in place before you embark on this journey could be the key to your success.

Also try to be really honest with other friends and family. Admit when you're struggling or finding things hard. If you have a bad day, phone a friend and tell them. We all need a helping hand sometimes, and there's nothing wrong with asking for support. It's what got me through some of my toughest moments.

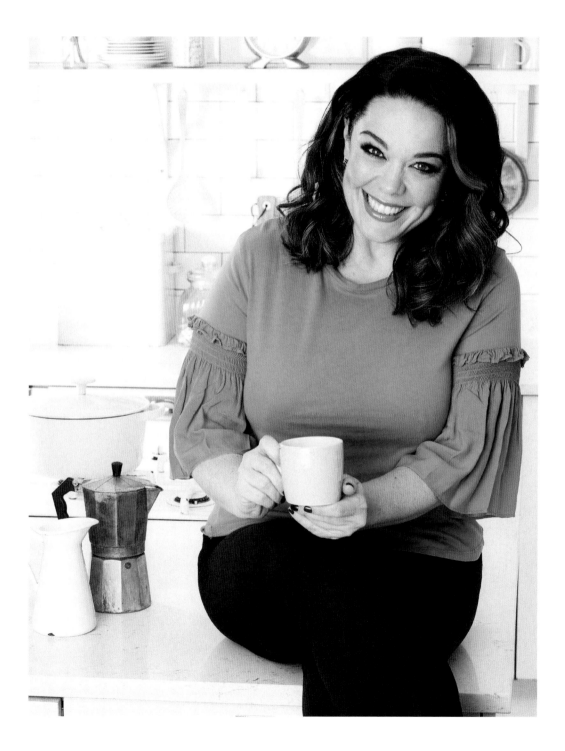

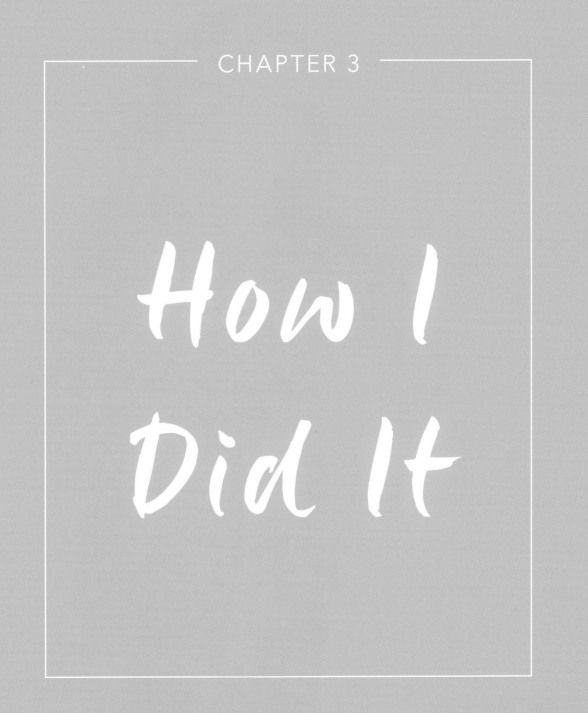

CHAPTER 3

How I
Did It

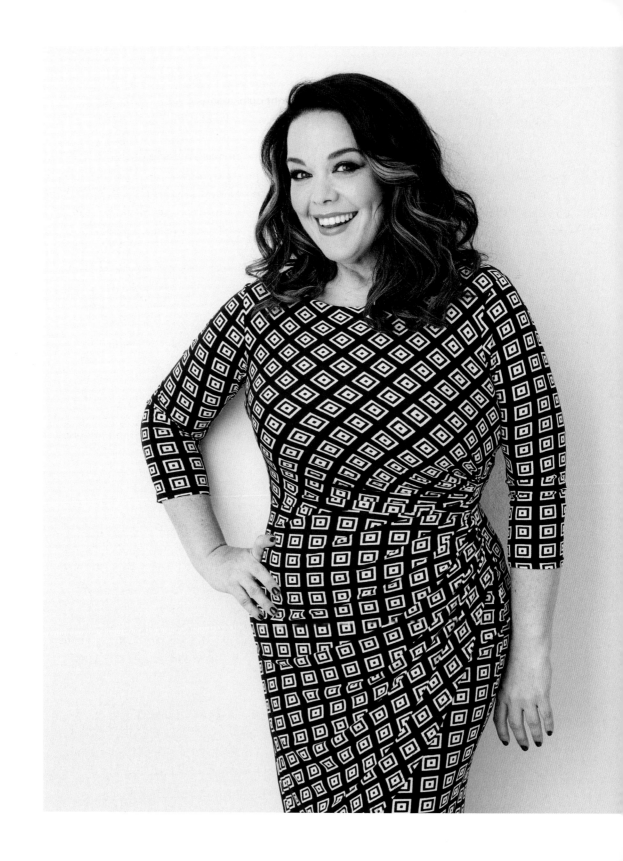

I've been asked a million times what my weight-loss 'light bulb' moment was – if there was a particular thing that flicked a switch and kick-started it – and the truth is that I had several.

Losing my mum to cancer in 2012, when she was only fifty-seven, was a massive catalyst. It changed the way I viewed the world and made me take a step back and really look at life. I lost my mum and my poppa, my mum's dad, within seventeen months. Poppa was my world, and losing both of them completely devastated me and made me hold the rest of my loved ones closer to me than ever. It also made me think about my own mortality and how many years I may have left.

A couple of years ago, doctors thought my dad had prostate cancer, and I completely spiralled. I was absolutely terrified. Thankfully, after tests, he was given the all-clear, but he was then diagnosed with type 2 diabetes, which was another wake-up call for me.

I knew that my size also put me at high risk of developing the disease. Did I want to follow in his footsteps and become a statistic?

No! But if I carried on the way I was, it was almost inevitable.

Type 2 diabetes has more than doubled in the UK over the last twenty years. If the current trend continues:
- 1 in 3 people will be obese by 2034
- 1 in 10 will develop type 2 diabetes

I went to visit my dad in hospital one day when he was being treated. He was on a ward of twenty-one men, all with type 2 diabetes. Some of them had lost limbs or gone blind as a result of the illness. Once it sets in, it can have a domino effect. Scarily, it's not an old person's disease, either. Some of the other men on the ward were young, and that put the fear of God into me.

I needed to be frightened into doing something about my weight, and that was the moment that did it. I'd looked in the mirror all my life and seen myself as this girl who was fat and funny and had a great career. That's who I was. But I looked at those men on the ward and realized that's how I would most likely end up.

I think I'm quite a unique case because, aside from the health issues and the odd dig from the press, my weight really wasn't bothering me that much. I didn't hate myself and nor did I wish I were thin. I'd resigned myself to the fact that I was always going to be fat. I'd justified it to myself over the years and allowed myself to accept that I'd always be that way. I didn't even think I could be the person I am now.

There can be so many reasons for being overweight. Emotional triggers play a massive part, and I was at my biggest when Mum's tumour came back for a second time. I honestly didn't know if I could survive without her.

I was so unhappy and lacking in energy, I was living on takeaways. I wanted to push all my feelings down, and every time I was upset I grabbed food. I never knew when to put the lid on the marmalade. I was scared that, when I did, the lid would come off my feelings instead and I wouldn't be able to cope.

They say don't keep putting food out for a puppy, because it doesn't know when to stop eating, and that was me. I didn't know when I was full, because I was emotionally starving.

We're not like cars, where you have no choice but to stop putting more petrol in once they're full. We can keep on eating when we're full, so we have to self-regulate, which I wasn't terribly good at. If you've got to the point where you're obese, you've been putting £30 worth of fuel in your tank when it really only needs a fiver's worth. You've got to stop at some point. Or the reality is, you could become very unwell.

We've all heard the saying 'break down to break through', and that's how it happened for me.

So if you're feeling crap right now? Great! Let's see that as a positive thing, because it means you're probably open to change.

I had some of my lowest moments just before I started losing weight. There were times when I felt like I was at the end of my tether. I needed to lose weight so I could stay well. But could I do it?

I felt so stuck. Someone might as well have dumped me in a massive bucket of concrete and let it set fast around my feet. I didn't think I'd ever be able to move forward. It felt like such a massive task. I had so much weight to lose. At the very least ten stone, which is a whole person! But, by letting myself go to that dark place, I found light.

If you feel like you can't do it right now, that's fine. Honestly. Don't try to push those feelings down. Acknowledge them, and then tell them to sod off.

There's light at the other end of this long tunnel, but only you can get yourself there. No one is going to be behind you, pushing you all the way.

I had to take responsibility for myself. One hundred per cent. And so do you.

I get messages all the time from people, and the main questions I get asked are:

- How did you do it?
- What are your secrets?
- Can you help me?
- Can you give me some of your willpower?

In this book I'm giving you the tools. But no one else can use them for you.

I CAN'T GIVE YOU WILLPOWER.

There isn't a day that goes by now when I'm not asked, 'How can I get your willpower?'

You have to find your own. It only exists when you want it inside out and back to front.

NO, I HAVEN'T HAD A GASTRIC BAND FITTED!

I've lost count of the number of times over the past year I've been asked if I've had a gastric band fitted. Some people still think I've had one. My skin removal surgeon, Dr Rob Winterton, has said categorically that he wouldn't have been able to physically operate on me even if I'd wanted one, so he is my absolute proof. He even asked me if I wanted him to take a photo while I was on the operating table to prove there was no band there, but I thought that was a step too far.

I've also been accused of taking something called raspberry ketones. I don't even know what they are or what they do! I refused to do any of those quick fixes. People don't want to believe I've lost all this weight through sheer hard work, but I have.

I had to effectively give myself a 'virtual gastric band' really early on in the diet. Your stomach doesn't want to be a watermelon, it wants to be a grapefruit! So I had to train mine to need less food. Now you're going to do the same. You may experience some hunger pangs initially, but your body will soon adjust as your stomach shrinks. I get full so quickly now, I can't physically eat any more than I need.

MS MOTIVATOR

Lots of things keep me motivated on a daily basis, but I'd say the most important ones for me are:

- how happy I wake up feeling every day
- my wardrobe!

Early on, it was the promise of those two things that kept me going.

I used to go on holiday with my mates every year, and none of my friends are above a size 14. At my biggest I was a size 28, and at my (previous) smallest a size 20, so I was always the one who made the biggest splash in the pool.

Every time the plane landed at our holiday destination, I'd panic about a luggage carousel moment. I'd think to myself, 'What the hell is going to happen if my suitcase goes missing? What will I wear?' My friends would have been able to borrow each other's clothes. Not me. And I've never seen plus size shops abroad, so I would have been completely stuck. I'd have had to wash the same pair of knickers and dress to wear every day.

Now, when I go on holiday with friends I can share clothes with them. I cannot tell you how good that feels. One of my friends came to stay recently and she forgot her pyjamas. She was able to borrow a pair of mine – and she didn't need to borrow an elasticated belt to hold the bottoms up!

Another clothing-related moment that really sticks out for me was when my friend Kate got married a few years ago. I was one of seven bridesmaids, and I had to have a different dress to all the other girls. They were all in these pretty, sleeveless numbers, while I was being held in by a giant cummerbund and thick sleeves.

When my friend Flossie asked me to be her maid of honour, I was worried I'd have to go through the humiliation of the fittings all over again. But thankfully I'd already started losing weight. By the time the last fitting rolled around I had to have my size 12 dress taken in! Flossie and I both stood in the bridal shop crying our eyes out.

Flossie sent me such a beautiful card afterwards, saying how proud she is of me and how wonderful it is to see how happy I've become. That meant the absolute world to me.

I'm much more experimental with clothes now. I want to wear everything! When I wore a jumpsuit on *Loose Women* I was so happy I screamed, and it still makes me smile when I think about it.

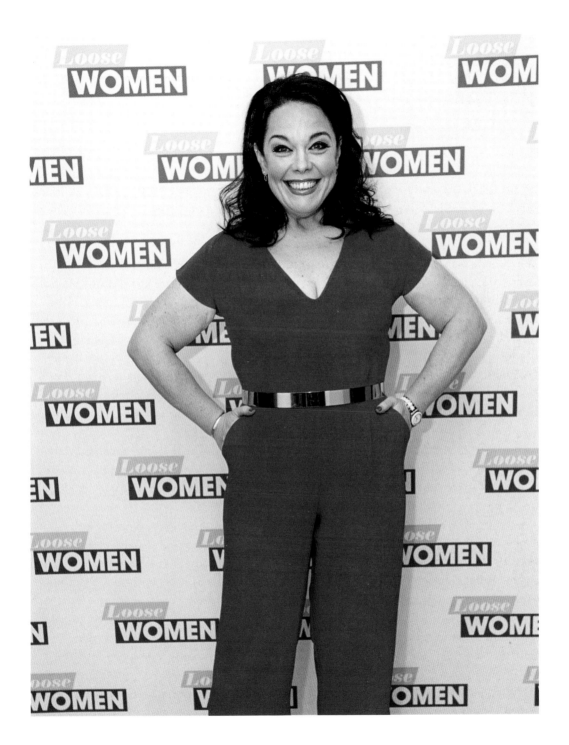

Before, I spent my life hiding behind baggy, black and dark-coloured clothes, but now I love colour. My world is brighter in every way.

Wearing nice clothes is the biggest natural high for me. I can't explain how good it feels. I never used to wear trainers. I felt I had to wear heels all the time, because otherwise I looked dumpy, but now I love flat shoes.

These days, I can go shopping with my mates and not have to go to the plus size shops on my own after they've gone home laden with bags of lovely clothes.

I appreciate every single moment. And so will you.

When a friend of mine who was also on a diet fitted into a pair of jeans she loved, she danced around her bedroom with joy. All of those moments help get you to where you want to be. They keep you striving.

Things changed massively for me when I posted a photo of myself on holiday in Singapore. I'd gone away travelling for six weeks and I put the photo on Twitter in March 2016. It's just a nice holiday snap where I'm standing at the front of a boat smiling, and I didn't think anything of it. Then all of a sudden I seemed to be on the cover of every magazine, and my phone was ringing off the hook with people asking how I'd lost weight.

I'd already done an intensive boot camp at that point and I'd seen an immediate change – hence why I recommend you begin with my 8-Day Kick-Start (see page 109)! Once I'd lost a bit of weight and seen that what I was doing was working, I stepped things up. I was doing it for me and no one else. I hadn't really told anyone, which is why people were surprised when this photo emerged. All I'd said to my family was that I'd started going to the gym. They'd probably thought, 'Yeah, right.'

I started to teach myself about dieting, because I wanted to go back to basics. I got googling and soon realized the weight-loss world was a minefield, and there was so, so much conflicting advice. I read and read and read. I used my brain, figured out what would work and what was a lot of tosh. And I set myself boundaries. I decided that my common sense and my body would let me know what was best for me, and I turned out to be right.

That Singapore photo means so much to me now. It's a record of the moment my life truly changed. The positive reaction I had from others was so amazing that it spurred me on to lose even more weight.

I was away on holiday for another three and a half weeks after I posted that picture, and when I got home I was invited to go on *Loose Women* as a guest. After that, things went even crazier, and people were saying such nice things about how I looked. Their comments motivated me so much. The reaction was so overwhelming, and I started to feel great about myself.

In fact, I felt better with every day that passed. It was like some kind of awakening.

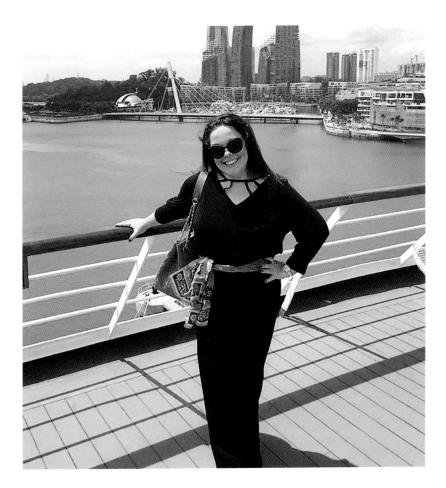

Going travelling was one of the things that had the biggest effect on me. It really broadened my horizons. In the far-flung places I visited, I couldn't get fish, chips and mushy peas for £3. I was so lucky that I got to see new parts of the world and embrace other cultures, and that had a huge impact on me.

Instead of swallowing food, I swallowed the world.

If I have down days now, I look back at the photos of where I've been. And they lift me.

My mum always told me that I should learn something new every day – and I did; when I travelled. I also realized what mattered. I'd been living in a safe little bubble, holding myself back from doing things because of my weight. I'd used it as an excuse.

But once I lost weight, I no longer felt I had to hide. I began to feel like I could do anything.

I was always the girl who had to ask for an extender belt on a plane. People used to panic when they saw me walking towards them, thinking they were going to have to spend the journey squashed next to me. Now I have so much extra length on the belt. On trains, I used to have to rest my boobs on the table in front of me, and I was so uncomfortable all the time. But I don't take up excess space any more.

Seeing the world opened my eyes. It meant I had to throw off my security blanket and embrace everything around me.

Photos have been a big part of my weight loss generally. I have an app on my phone called Timehop, which shows me pictures from the same day in previous years. If you don't have it, download it now. It's like therapy for me. Seeing old pictures gives me a kick up the arse to go to the gym!

When I look back now through all the photos of me at different sizes, it's like I'm a set of Russian dolls – getting smaller over time, as each layer of excess weight is lifted away.

KEEP IT REAL

I don't want to put a downer on things but I do want to give you the tools for the hard times as well as the good. I need you to be prepared for what I call reverse motivation. You may have mornings when you wake up and don't feel as positive as you'd like to, or you feel like you've stalled. I call these 'impatience pangs'. You may find yourself acting like a spoilt brat, who wants to be slim NOW! Sorry, it doesn't work that way.

I hit a big wall about six weeks after I started my diet. I'd initially seen this massive change in my body. But after the excitement and novelty had worn off, I suddenly realized I still wasn't anywhere near the top of the mountain, and I had a steep climb ahead of me yet.

Could I carry on when I knew how much effort I'd need to put in? Or was it simpler to turn around and slide back down the mountain, grabbing a tube of Pringles on the way?

Thankfully, I was so determined that I stuck with it.

At those times when I plateaued, or if I felt like things weren't moving along, I would go for a monster walk to clear out the cobwebs. The boost to my cardio always made me feel so much better – both physically and emotionally – and then I was able to carry on. Being honest enabled me to self-motivate. The old me would have thought, 'It's so much easier to go to the pub than for a walk,' and I'd make so many excuses to justify why it was okay to do that.

Then I got real.

By using my Honesty Diary I began to work out what my weakest moments were, and I would recommend you do the same. After you've been writing in your diary for a few weeks, look back and see if you can spot any patterns that have revealed themselves along the way.

Did you snack in front of the TV because it was a Saturday and you 'deserved' a treat?

Do you find you struggled more at weekends when your days weren't as regimented, or you were seeing friends or going out for family lunches?

Maybe your diary shows that certain times of day are trickier for you?

Did you often want to reach for a sugary snack to combat the mid-afternoon slump?

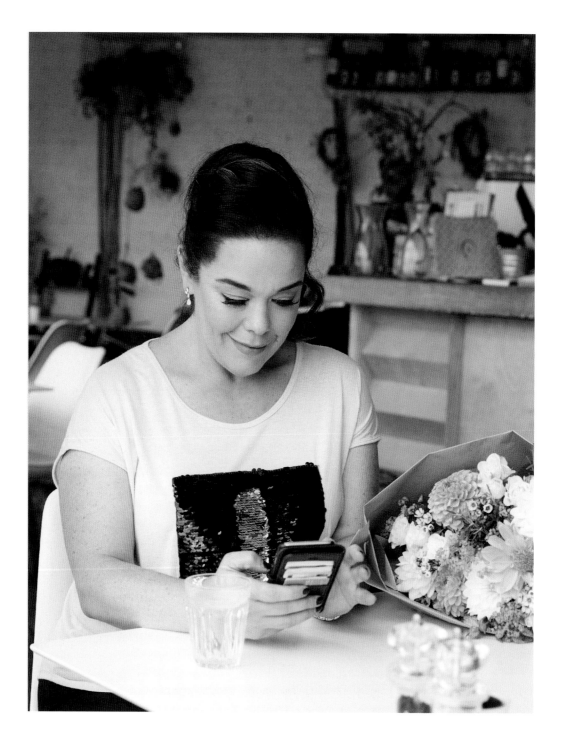

Or can you identify any emotional triggers that might have caused you to eat – or want to eat – things you shouldn't? Look at the moments when you struggled and think about what else was happening at that point. Did you have a stressful meeting at work? Were your kids playing up? Were you upset or tired for any particular reason? Once you figure out those triggers that put your diet at risk, you'll be much more in control of them – and then you can learn how to protect yourself when you know they're coming up.

This strategy certainly worked for me. I learned so much about myself thanks to everything I put down in my Honesty Diary.

My progress has been like the Grand National. Some of the jumps were really hard. But when you cross the finish line, you will never have another feeling like it.

My weight loss certainly wasn't all plain sailing. I looked at myself naked in the mirror after I'd lost quite a lot of weight and I still didn't like what I saw. I don't know if I thought I'd magically look amazing, but it wasn't what I was expecting. Instead of thinking about how far I'd come, I thought about how far I still had to go, and I felt very disheartened.

I remember lying in the bath one time, crying. My boobs were banging around like canoes, and my body was all so desperately loose. I lay there pulling at my rolls of fat. It was horrendous.

I know so many people who have had that awful bath moment. I wouldn't wish it on my worst enemy. It's only people who have experienced it who can properly sympathize.

I found sanctuary online. I discovered there were other people in the same position as I was, which is why I always try to be there for people now. I've lived through the pain. I know how it feels.

Weeks six, seven and eight are when most people fall off the weight-loss wagon and turn to comfort food. That will be the point when you may feel a bit defeated and wonder if you're supposed to always be overweight.

You're not.

You are in control of your climb.

While one week you may not feel like you've lost any weight, you could end up taking a big leap the following week. Even if you can't see the evidence of the weight melting away, things are going on behind the scenes. Your body is working, and it's quietly getting used to its new regime.

Trust your body. It knows what works for you, and it will support you. You may have felt let down by your body in the past and angry at it for not being perfect. Or you may have suffered from illness and blamed it for hampering your ability to lose weight. But I will say this:

IF YOU'RE EATING WELL AND EXERCISING ENOUGH, YOU WILL LOSE WEIGHT.

You can't not – it's basic maths and science. And you certainly shouldn't put any on. (If you do, despite eating well and exercising, then I recommend you see your doctor. In particular, ask them to check your thyroid.) But if your health is fine, the only way you'll put weight on is if you go back to your old ways. And that is not something you will do, right? When it comes to exercise, you have to learn to enjoy the burn. Those physical reactions mean your body is changing for good.

MINDFULNESS

Another thing that really helped me when things felt overwhelming was the technique of mindfulness. If I needed some time out, I'd take it.

I'd give myself ten minutes just sitting in silence, remembering why I'd started out on this journey. Then I'd fast-forward in my head to the finale of my weight-loss film, and picture my happy ending.

I used to be the worst culprit for not taking time out for myself. But now I have a newfound appreciation of just how important it is.

Even if it's just a couple of minutes of closing your eyes on a bus or train journey and taking a few deep breaths, it all helps. I'm not suggesting you strike a yoga pose in the middle of the aisle, but do what you can to relax.

We don't do it enough.

I'll also watch movies (without food treats!) or read a book to distract myself if my head gets a bit noisy. I used to reach for the wine, but all-new Lisa doesn't do that.

Which brings me to my next point . . .

BYE BYE BOOZE

One of the biggest changes I made to my life right at the beginning of my weight-loss journey was cutting out alcohol. And I hate to say it, but if you want this diet to work its best for you, then you should consider doing the same. Booze is not a slimmer's friend.

I used to be the queen of Malbec. I'd drink it when I was happy, when I was down and wanted a bit of a lift, or as a reward after a long day.

Did I drink more after my mum passed away?

God, yes.

Did it make the pain go away?

No. It made me feel worse the following day when I had hangover depression and knew that my mum was still never coming back. It was the world's worst comfort blanket.

I was a classic binge drinker on nights out, and I could happily drink two bottles over the course of a long evening. Things couldn't be more different now. I haven't had a drop for over two years. And I don't miss it one bit.

I'm certainly not saying everyone should give up drinking forever, just because I have. It's totally up to each individual. But I will say that for the duration of this diet, I urge you to:

PUT THE BOTTLE DOWN!

Not only does alcohol contain a lot of empty calories, it also weakens your emotional defences, so the chances are you'll end up mindlessly snacking or reaching for a burger or a kebab at the end of the night.

Then there's hangover hunger. How many of us have eaten a week's worth of calories in a single session the day after a big drinking sesh?

There wasn't enough food in the world to satisfy my hunger when I had a post-booze sugar craving. And, funnily enough, it wasn't apples and carrots I gorged on. It was crisps, heavily buttered toast and takeaways. I was drawn to anything beige and loaded with fat.

On a typical hangover day I could easily eat a thick-crust margarita pizza laden with mozzarella and pineapple, a side of chips and gravy, all washed down with two litres of non-diet Sprite.

These days, I associate drinking alcohol with being at my absolute biggest, and it's that association that has helped me to give up. There's one photo of me at an event wearing a red and black dress, when I was out for the third night on the trot. I look so bloated and ill – I don't ever want to look that bad again.

I hid my hangovers really well. Any time I was feeling terrible, I hit the bravado button. No one would have known from my painted-on smile that all I wanted to do was climb under a duvet and stay there all day. I became a master at pretending I was A-okay.

Giving up drinking was essential to my weight loss. For me it had to be all or nothing. Even if I'd cut right down and just had the occasional drink every couple of weeks, it would have had a huge effect on how quickly I lost weight.

It would take me a few days now to consume the number of calories I used to drink on a single night out. And that's before you include the late-night drunken eating. There's no way I would sit and eat three bars of chocolate at once, these days. But on nights out I used to drink the equivalent of that in wine, and then some.

I don't mean to sound preachy (I know there's nothing more boring), but nowadays I love getting up and feeling good every morning. I used to hate it when I woke up and only dared to open one eye at a time, so I could test how bad my hangover was. If I had a dry mouth and a pounding headache, I knew my day was going to be a write-off.

Now, I'm always alert for work. I have tons of energy. And, instead of diving straight for the kitchen, to eat everything in sight, I very often do exercise first thing. I know, I'm shocked too!

I have so much more time now that I don't drink, because I don't spend days hung-over. I spoil myself with time instead.

And if people say I'm boring? I laugh it off. I have never felt less boring.

I was the girl who would fall through the door hammered at 3 a.m. Now I'm the girl who's in the gym at 6.30 a.m.

When do you think I was happier? Go on, take a guess!

The honest truth is that now I get my highs from doing exercise classes. Try it! You might love it, too. Or you could put on the Gipsy Kings and salsa around your kitchen. I defy you not to smile while you're doing it.

Luckily, leaving the boozy nights behind was pretty easy for me. Because once I put my mind to something, I tend to go for it (no wonder my bad habits were all super-sized). But I had to get to the point where it was something I *wanted* to do.

It was the same with dieting. I've been offered so much money to record weight-loss DVDs over the years, but I didn't have the will to do it. And achieving rapid weight loss by not eating, and then piling it all back on again within weeks, wasn't for me. I didn't want to deceive people in order to make a quick buck. If I was going to talk publicly about losing weight, I wanted it to be in an honest and real way that was achievable for other people.

It took me a long time to look like this, and I know that I have to eat the right things and keep my exercise up if I want to stay looking like this.

The reality is that I won't ever be able to go back to eating like I used to. Unless I want to pile on the pounds again.

For me, it was never going to be a case of going on a diet and then going back to eating cheesy chips every lunchtime.

THIS IS A LIFESTYLE FOR ME, NOT A TEMPORARY FIX.

It's become as much a part of my life as having a shower and getting dressed each morning.

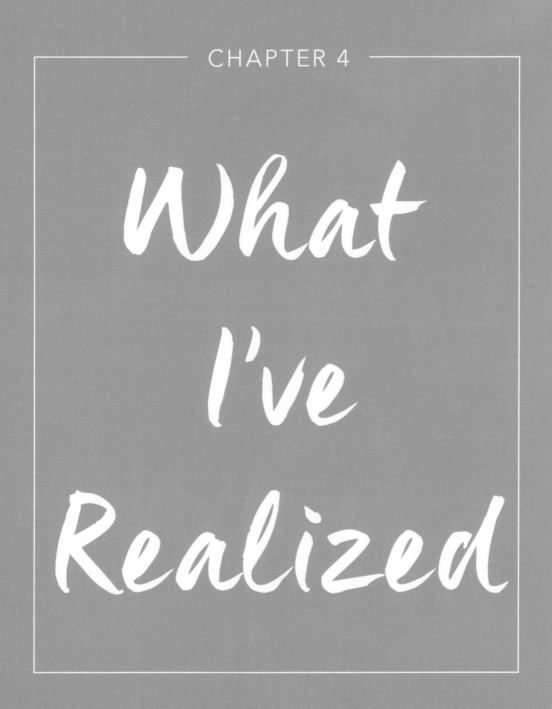

CHAPTER 4

What I've Realized

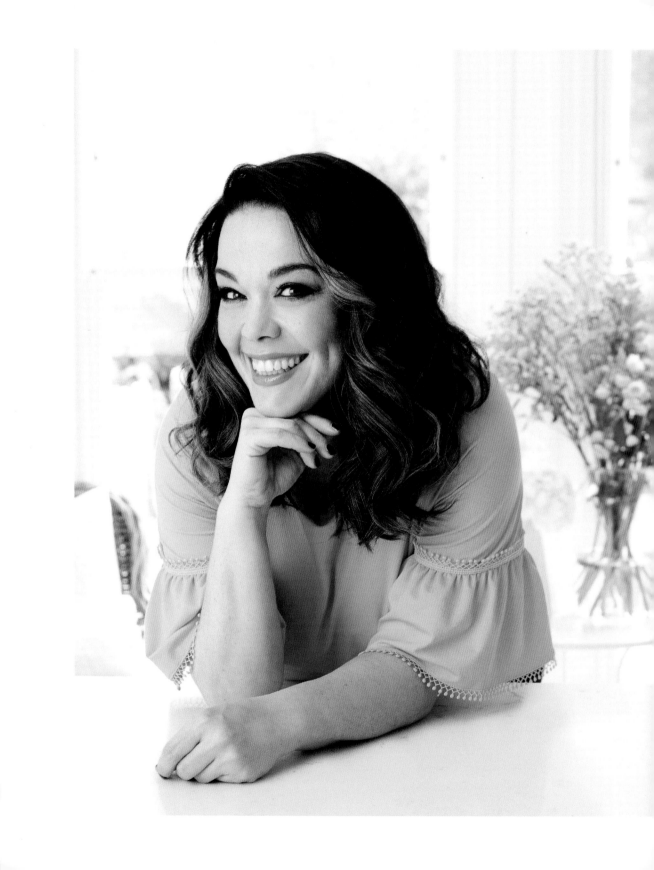

Looking back now, I can clearly see that I had to get to the point where I wanted to take good care of myself. For a long time I'd had such a battering from the press that I didn't think I deserved to like how I looked. I was happy in a lot of ways, but not as happy as I could have been. And certainly not as happy as I am now.

I find it so hard to look back at my old overweight self – and I do struggle with putting 'old Lisa' to bed at times – but I'm done with her. My weight is still a big talking point for people. I have paparazzi wanting to take pictures of me all the time, because everyone is waiting for me to put the weight back on so they can run a story about how I've failed. But they'll be waiting a long time.

I am aware of what I put in my mouth every day. I've seen women slim down to a size 8, and then put it all back on again. I am one hundred per cent determined I'm not going to do that.

A friend of mine said to me recently, 'Do you think you'll always be on a diet?' I said, 'No, but I'll forever be mindful of what I eat, and I'll always go for healthy options.' That's my reality. Feeling this good every day makes me a million times happier than any cake ever could. I don't want anything to ever take this feeling away from me.

So if anyone else asks, I'm not on a 'diet' diet now. This is just me!

PRACTICE MAKES PERFECT

Losing weight takes practice. The more you practise dieting, the better you'll get at it. The first couple of days are always the hardest, but crack those and then you'll be flying.

There will be tough moments along the way – believe me, I know – but keep writing in your Honesty Diary and reflecting on your progress to get you through. I documented everything: the good, the bad and the ugly. It helped me remember why I was doing this in the first place.

We know that cravings aren't always down to hunger. Sometimes they can be negative feelings that you want to push down with biscuits or cakes. Then, once you've eaten them, you're so annoyed with yourself that you try to quash the guilt by eating even more. The way to stop the cycle is to acknowledge those feelings, instead of trying to ignore them, by – drum roll! – writing it all down.

It really is now or never. People ask why I waited until I was thirty-nine to lose weight, and I don't have a clever answer. It was finally the right time for me to rebuild myself. Now it's your turn.

MY DIET:
BEFORE AND AFTER

Warning: You may be shocked!

MY DIET BEFORE	MY DIET AFTER
Breakfast Four slices of white toast with loads of butter Coco Pops with full-fat milk Coffee with sugar	**Breakfast** Hot water and lemon Porridge with honey
Lunch Cheese and onion toasty with fries Can of Tango	**Lunch** Butternut squash and coriander soup with oatcakes
Dinner Mushroom tagliatelle with garlic bread Tiramisu Bottle of Malbec wine Non-diet fizzy drinks	**Dinner** Garlic and chilli cod with roasted spinach and cauliflower
Supper Two toasted crumpets and jam	**Desperate measures** Almonds or plain cashews Fruit Coffee with a splash of almond milk
Snacks between meals Crisps Sandwiches Bars of chocolate Non-diet fizzy drinks Bowls of cereal	

MY BIG OPS

It's been well documented that I've had two major operations to remove excess skin since I lost weight. But it wasn't a decision I took lightly. Once I had decided to go for it, I knew I had to be one hundred per cent truthful about it. Surgery wasn't ever something I was going to try and hide from anyone.

I first decided I was going to go down the surgery route in December 2016. I'd already lost a lot of weight, and things felt like they were slotting into place. But the looser my skin became, the harder and more painful I found it to exercise. I felt like I was carrying a giant bag of spuds around with me the whole time.

Everything started to hurt, and when I tried to bend down, my bib (the bit of fat that hangs down off your stomach) got in the way. No amount of exercise was going to remedy that.

I wanted to have my legs, groin and a fleur-de-lis done, which is also known as a lower-body lift. It involves excess skin being removed from the abdominal area, and it's such a big op that people have died from complications whilst having it done.

The only surgery I'd ever had before was a tonsillectomy when I was fifteen, so I definitely felt that I was putting myself in a very dangerous situation if I went ahead. I would be on an operating table for six hours, and it would put my organs under a lot of pressure. Rather more serious than having a tooth out.

I mulled things over for ages. I'd stopped drinking and smoking, and I'd lost a ton of weight. So health-wise I knew it was the best possible time for me to have the op.

But was it worth the risk?

After approximately a million discussions with my mates, I decided to go for it.

I went for a consultation at the Spire Hospital in Manchester, and before you could say, 'You're just going to feel a little prick,' my operation date was set.

I tried my best to be relaxed about it. But the closer the day came, the more anxious I felt and there were times when I almost pulled out. I got it into my head that keeping myself really busy in the lead-up would mean I didn't have time to think about the upcoming surgery as much.

Lots of people knew I was planning to have it done. But I was also trying to keep the actual date quiet, so that I didn't have added pressure. The last thing I wanted was paps taking photos of me as I hobbled out of the hospital.

The week before the operation I had the most horrific dreams. I saw myself being carried out of my house in a body bag, and all sorts. Weirdly, I kept worrying my heart wouldn't be strong enough to handle the procedure, even though I knew my body was in fact the fittest it had ever been. Ironically, my heart was actually under a lot more strain when I was desperately overweight.

I was born with a heart murmur and I had tests every year until I was cleared of the condition at seven years old. My mum was quite neurotic about it and she was always telling me to be careful, which had a knock-on effect on me. I'd not thought about it for years. But because I was panicking about the operation, it suddenly all came back to the surface and began bubbling away again.

Medically, I was in the best place I could possibly be – and the human body can withstand an incredible amount of pressure. My surgeon had effectively rebuilt someone after they'd had a motorcycle accident. He's a genius, so I felt completely confident about that side of things. But emotionally, I was a mess.

The day before the operation, I went into our pre-show meeting at *Loose Women* and the other girls started asking me about the op, not knowing I was booked to go into hospital the following morning. I suddenly started thinking, 'This time tomorrow, I could be dead.' It was terrifying, and I went into panic mode. When I got home that day, I started crying and couldn't stop. I knew that the surgeon and the anaesthetist were some of the best in the business, and I was in safe hands. But it was still so scary.

I'd never felt fear like it before, and I haven't since.

I was so worried about my little nephews: Jakey, six, and Joshua, three. How would they react if anything happened to me?

They knew I was going into hospital. I'd told them that Auntie Lee Lee was getting a new belly button, so that they wouldn't worry.

On the morning of the operation I was a wreck. I was physically shaking, but the staff at the hospital were so comforting and understanding. I was filming my documentary, *Lisa Riley's Baggy Body Club*, at the time and when the people working on the show saw how terrified I was, they genuinely didn't expect me to get on that operating table.

When I watched the footage back I could see the fear that was in my eyes. I didn't realize at the time quite how frightened I was, but it was very clear from the look on my face. I don't think I allowed myself to acknowledge just how bad I was feeling, and I did everything I could to distract myself.

Thankfully, before I knew it, I was gowned up and being given my anaesthetic by a brilliant man called Patch. And then there was no going back . . .

. . . and that's the last thing I remember clearly.

I came round after the operation but it's all very hazy because of the medication I was on. One of the scariest things for me was the reaction I had to one of the painkillers. It affected me so badly I started hallucinating. I was convinced one-eyed worms were coming out of the curtains and trying to eat me. It was like Alice in Wonderland meets Freddy Krueger. That painkiller was replaced with another one – straight away!

The following day, I was so relieved it was all over. And so happy that I'd gone for it. I knew I'd done the right thing because it had worked, even if I wasn't feeling my perkiest.

Dr Rob Winterton chopped 15 lbs – more than a stone! – of skin off me during the first operation, which was just incredible.

People always ask me how painful it was, and I can't be anything but (you guessed it) honest. Pain is graded out of eight in hospital, and I would say it was very much at the top of the range. For a long time afterwards the word 'comfortable' wasn't in my vocabulary.

I guess my first operation gave me the confidence to have the second one. But I was still very nervous about that one, too. I had a gap of ten weeks between the two operations, and the second one concentrated on my boobs and arms. I was lucky that I still had a lot of tissue left in my boobs, so Dr Winterton was able to rebuild them without implants. He's a genuine miracle worker.

I suffered with seromas both times – where fluid builds up under your skin – which was very painful and set my recovery back a lot. I blame some of it on moving house so soon after the first operation. I was lifting boxes and bookcases, and I probably shouldn't have been lifting even a bottle of water at that point. I thought it was a positive thing, because I was moving around a lot. But I tried to do too much too quickly, and it backfired, leading to complications.

I wasn't able to exercise at all, and I hated it. I was petrified of putting on weight again and it messed with my head. By now I was used to moving around constantly, yet all I could do was lie on the sofa like a sloth while the seromas healed. I felt like a caged animal. But I had no choice other than to rest and focus on getting better. Looking back, it was a bad time.

I'd learned my lesson after the first operation, and so I really listened to everyone after operation number two. I gave myself some proper time to recover, and as soon as Rob gave me the green light to get back to the gym, I was there.

I experienced some tough and emotional moments. But once the bandages came off and I saw the results, it all felt so worth it.

The scars are still healing, but I'm delighted at how well and how fast it's all happening. I've got Arnica gel that I rub in using circular movements, and it's working amazingly well.

I've got no regrets whatsoever.

I am done with surgery now. If I were to have anything else done, it would be what I call my 'bra cupcake', which is the fat that hangs over my bra straps at the back. It really bugs me but, in the grand scheme of things, it's not a huge deal, and it's something I am going to target through exercise instead.

It's so easy to get caught in the never-ending trap of fixing one thing after another.

Let's face it, who doesn't want to improve how they look?

But I was once the girl who cried as she pulled at her body like Play-Doh. So I'm very thankful about how far I've come.

I was a very extreme case. Unless you have a very large amount of weight to lose – like I did – the chances are you won't suffer from loose, saggy skin.

In my opinion surgery should only be considered as a last resort. If you can get back into shape without it, fantastic. But I guess it is good to be aware that the option is there for people who truly find that nothing else will work.

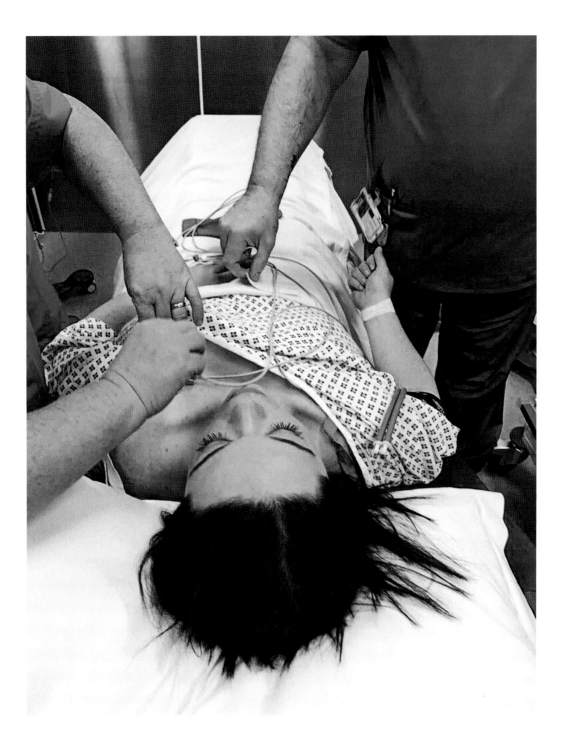

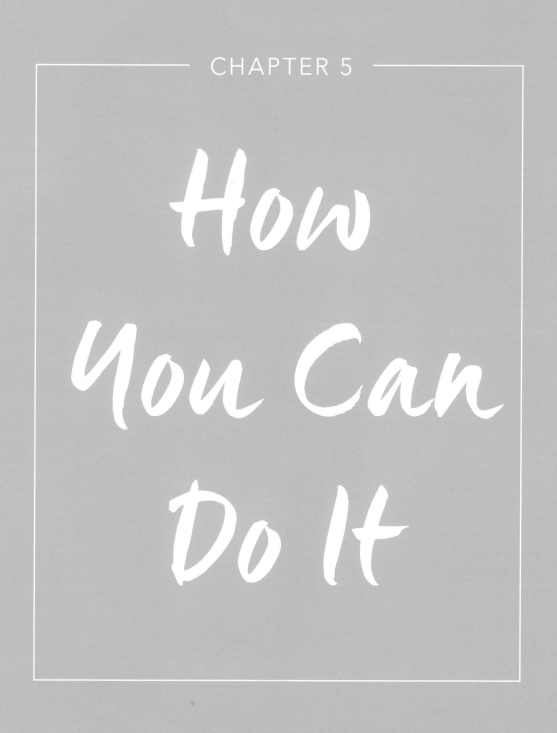

CHAPTER 5

How You Can Do It

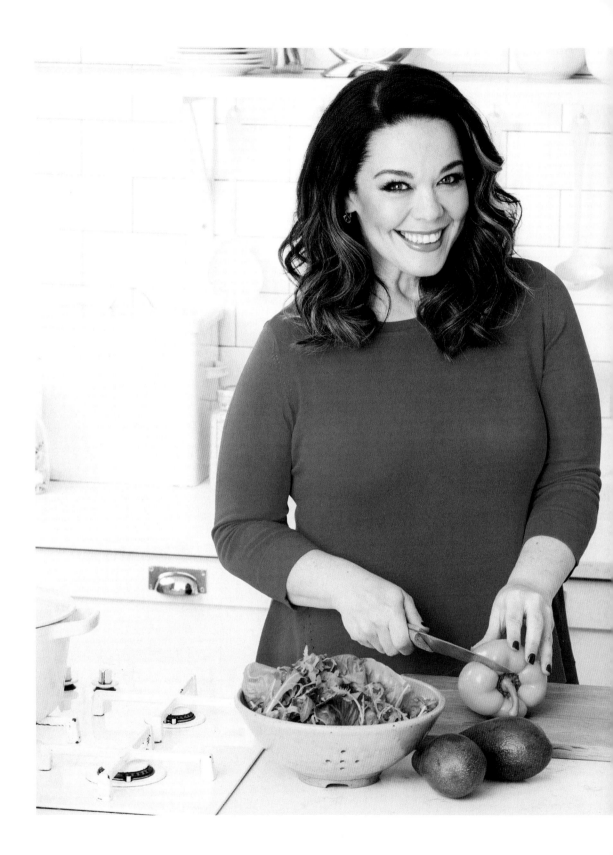

First and foremost, stop making excuses! I don't want to hear them.

'I'll start again tomorrow.'

'This little bit won't hurt.'

'It's my time of the month.'

I've heard them all. Every time you go to tell yourself a fib or make an excuse, stop yourself and write it down in your Honesty Diary. You'll be shocked at how many times you do it in a single day.

If I can lose weight, so can you.

You can make all the excuses in the world, but the only person you'll be lying to is yourself. All those little fibs are self-sabotage that is stopping you from getting to where you want to be.

THINGS THAT COULD SCUPPER YOUR WEIGHT LOSS

These are the biggest pitfalls to watch out for. Avoid these and your weight-loss journey will be much smoother.

COMPARING YOURSELF TO OTHER PEOPLE

Most of us have got that one friend who can eat cakes, sweets and biscuits and not put on weight. That doesn't mean *you* can. If you keep asking yourself, 'Why can't I do that?' you'll only hold yourself back.

I was very realistic when I was losing weight that I wasn't ever going to be giving Kate Moss sleepless nights. I didn't pick up fashion magazines and kid myself I was going to look like a supermodel, because I'm not delusional. Nor did I ever set out to look like the girls in the gym adverts, because that's just not my body type. I didn't want to be 'perfect', I just wanted to be the best possible version of myself. You can't change who you are, but you can certainly improve on it.

Don't look at your slim mate and wonder why she can eat plates of creamy pasta and still wear skinny jeans. Some people are naturally small and they can eat what they like and not put on weight. But if you've bought this book, the chances are that isn't you.

A lot of slim people either watch what they eat, or they are used to eating healthily and stopping when they're full. They are also likely to be much more active – either doing a lot of exercise, or they may have a job that keeps them on their feet all day. It's rare to find someone who regularly devours entire cakes and still fits into a size 10. So ditch any unhelpful 'It's not fair' thoughts and get rid of unrealistic goals and comparisons.

The only person you should be competing with is the old version of yourself.

SCALES = FAILS

This is my mantra – and you may want it to become yours, too.

I'll weigh myself every now and again to keep an eye on things, but I'm not a slave to the scales. You can tell if you've lost weight because your clothes – and common sense – will tell you, so don't hop on and off the scales ten times a day just in case you've lost half a pound. You'll only depress yourself.

When I had to be weighed ahead of my operations, it put me in a horrible mindset and left me feeling deflated. It can really set people back if they step on the scales and they've put on weight from one day to the next. But it could be the time of the month, or just that you need the loo! That weight will soon come off again.

You don't want to be sent spiralling into a pit of weight-gain doom if you discover you've gained a pound. You might decide none of your hard work is worth it, and give up. That's the time when you grab unhealthy self-help food.

On the flip side, if you step on the scales and see a good weight loss, you might get complacent and think, 'Great, I can go and have a bacon sandwich now.' And that's when it all goes to pot.

We're all smart enough to know for ourselves when we're losing weight and when we're not. Listen to your body. It's so clever. Your body knows what shape you should naturally be. The first time I started to see my natural shape I cried my eyes out.

I try not to talk too much about exactly how much I weigh now and how much I weighed before I started dieting, because the precise numbers are not the most important thing to me. I was a size 28 and now I'm a size 12. I know I've lost over twelve stone, and that's all I care about. All the bits in between were part of the journey.

If you compare ten people who all weigh the same, the chances are they won't look the same, because everyone's body is different. Eleven stone sits very differently on one person than it does on another. Body shape is affected by height, muscle mass and how your frame distributes weight. So many factors come into play.

I do a lot of exercise now. So if I stepped on the scales, I might weigh more than I did a couple of months ago, because of my increased muscle mass (since muscle weighs more than fat does). But yet I might look slimmer than I did, because now I'm more toned. If you want to check your weight every month or two, fine, but please don't hop on and off the pound counters every day.

Say it with me. Scales = fails!

ONE-UPPERS

We've all got that competitive friend who wants to do one better than you. If you've lost a pound, they've lost two. If you've been to Tenerife, they've been to 'Elevenerife'.

If you've got mates like this who are also on diets, by all means congratulate them if they tell you they've lost weight. But don't let it bother you if they lose more than you at any point. Focus on your own journey.

WORRYING ABOUT WHAT OTHER PEOPLE THINK

The only person you have something to prove to here is you. You shouldn't fret about trying to impress other people, or project a false image on social media with airbrushed photos.

Women post photos of their weight loss on my social media all the time, and I absolutely love it. But there are some who I know lost weight and then put it back on again. They're still posting out-of-date pictures of themselves in order to look good to other people. But who are they trying to kid? The people looking at your photos aren't the ones that matter. You are.

The harsh reality is that other people don't think about you half as much as you think they do. Sorry, but it's the truth. They may read your status or look at your picture but, within seconds, they've usually moved on to look at someone else's. So don't worry about convincing other people that you look great. Focus on yourself in the here and now, and with time you'll look even better than you do in the photos on your social media profile.

There's no point in trying to convince the world you're slim if you're not, because at the end of the day you'll still feel rubbish. And people have eyes, so the next time they see you in the supermarket they'll realize you've been trying to hoodwink them.

'GUILT-FREE' SHARING

Just because you're sharing food with someone, it doesn't mean it has no calories.

The same goes for eating standing up, and for picking at food out of a pan instead of eating it from a plate.

I'm telling it to you straight: it all counts!

FREE FOOD

Had a couple of canapés at a party?

Ate the free breakfast bar sample they were giving out at the train station?

It doesn't matter if food is free. It still has calories!

GRABBING ON THE GO

Like a good cub scout, be prepared! I spend half of my life on trains, and even though the snack choice in the buffet cart has got better, there are still only a couple of things that are healthy enough to fit in with my new lifestyle.

So instead of running on to a train with seconds to spare and grabbing a mayo-laden sandwich,

I always make sure I take my own food. Even if it means nipping to the supermarket and grabbing a salad and some prawns before I board.

It's the same when you fly. You know before you even look at a plane menu that it's going to be full of crisps, chocolate and toasted panini. So I strongly recommend you eat in the airport beforehand, and eat well.

To be a successful dieter you have to plan. You can't leave it to chance. It's complacency that will make you reach for a Snickers.

MAILING LISTS

Take yourself off all restaurant email mailing lists. If you're dieting, you do not need to hear about two-for-one pizza deals.

SMALL IS NOT ALWAYS BEAUTIFUL

Just because a cake is small does not make it okay. It's still a cake. Always remember Dionne Warwick. Walk on by.

GETTING BORED

If you eat the same thing every day, you'll get bored and be more likely to reach for unhealthy snacks or treats. Mix things up and be adventurous. See my recipes on pages 139–251.

DENIAL

I went out with a friend of mine the other day and she had a salad for lunch. She followed it up with a chocolate cake and a cappuccino with two sugars.

After we left she said to me, 'I can't wait to tell my husband I only had a salad for lunch.'

Need I say more?

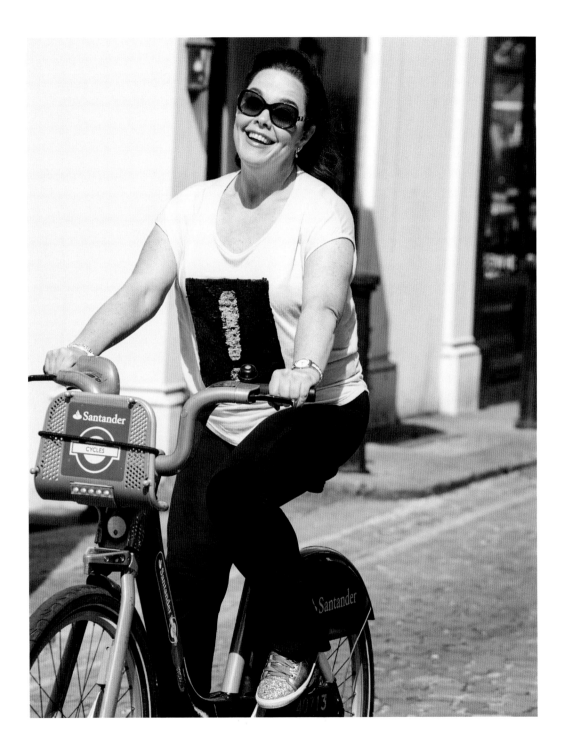

Back when I was big, I used to see comments like, 'Well, she got herself into that position.'

And you know what? I did. I bloody did. Nobody but me put food into my mouth. No one else filled up my supermarket trolley with biscuits and crisps, and no one else bought box after box of chocolates for me to mindlessly eat in front of the TV.

It took me a long time to realize that and to start being honest about it.

HOLIDAYS

Don't go on holiday thinking it's inevitable that you're going to put on a stone in two weeks. It doesn't have to be the case.

Be mindful. If you do come back bigger, remember that you did that to yourself.

It is possible to go on holiday and still eat healthily, especially if you've booked full-board or you're staying at an all-inclusive where there's usually a salad bar and lots of different options.

If you don't stick to your diet there's only one reason – because you decided not to.

THE 'ONE WON'T HURT' ATTITUDE

It will! Especially if you have lots of 'ones'.

It's a slippery slope. If you need to ask yourself, 'Does this count?' then the answer is, 'Yes, of course it does!'

COMFORT-TALKING

Comfort-eating is such a huge thing, but comfort-talking is just as dangerous. Telling yourself it's okay to eat something when you know it's not – that is where it all starts.

TAKING THAT FIRST STEP

Do you keep telling yourself you'll start tomorrow/Monday?

Well, the likelihood is you won't. You'll make more excuses instead and keep putting it off. It doesn't matter what you've already eaten today/this week. Start right here, right now.

Get your Honesty Diary out and get writing. Break the cycle.

You're either going to do it or you're not. If you don't want to lose weight, that's fine. But stop telling yourself and everyone else that you're going to. Because you'll only end up making yourself feel disheartened.

I get so many people messaging me saying they're at the end of their tether and they don't know how to change things. My answer is always the same:

JUST MAKE A START, AND THE REST WILL FOLLOW!

I don't promise that you will be a size 12 by next week. But in a year's time? Your body and your life could be totally different. You just have to take that first step. If you keep making excuses, you'll be in exactly the same position in five years' time, and life is too short for that.

Find your motivation – whether it's a picture of you at your slimmest, or someone who has lost a lot of weight (when people tell me they have a picture of me on their fridge as inspiration, I still find it unbelievable) – and know that you can get there. I've said it before and I'll say it again (and again and again): If I can do it, so can you!

Remember, if you don't change things, nothing ever changes. If you keep eating the same things and thinking in the same way, you'll get the same results. And you don't want to do that any more.

FOOD AMNESIA

I used to get food amnesia all the time. I'd eat something and then forget about it seconds later, as if it didn't happen. If I'd eaten it really quickly, or while on the go, I didn't seem to think it counted.

I'd get to the end of the day and I wouldn't have a clue about what or how much I'd put into my body. Now that I write everything down, I can't do that. It's all there, plain to see.

EATING LATE

Try not to do it! I have a personal cut-off time of 6.30 p.m. The way I see it, our bodies were designed to sleep when the sun goes down, not to process food.

And yes, those 'little' evening snacks in front of the TV do count. Busy yourself during ad breaks when all the tempting snack foods are being showcased. They can be a killer, so avoid them as much as possible.

Of course there may be days when you have no choice but to eat your evening meal a bit later. But if you eat enough for lunch and dinner, you shouldn't feel the need to pick late at night.

THINKING YOU'RE BEING HEALTHY WHEN YOU'RE NOT

Organic food is not automatically healthy. It may still contain sugar and fat. The same goes for gluten-free food.

Coeliacs have to eat gluten-free food because they are allergic and eating even the smallest amount of gluten is actually dangerous for them. But more and more people are turning to a gluten-free diet because they think it will help them lose weight. Here is a reality check: gluten-free products often have just as much sugar and fat in them as 'normal' foods. In some cases, because the gluten has been removed and replaced with something else, they'll have more!

I know someone who went on a gluten-free diet and put on half a stone in a month because she discovered the gluten-free cakes and biscuits in her local supermarket. She assumed that everything marked 'gluten free' was automatically healthy, so she was eating GF cookies like they were going out of fashion. She soon learned her lesson.

FOOD ALLERGIES

These days, you can pay for an intolerance test to find out if your body doesn't 'like' certain foods. I know people who've done that and then convinced themselves that if they cut out those specific foods, they'll instantly lose a ton of weight. I know they want an easy answer, but that's not it.

If not eating certain foods genuinely makes you feel better health-wise, great. But don't think that just because you've been told you react badly to tomatoes, you'll lose stones by cutting them out.

ASSUMING BEING VEGETARIAN/VEGAN IS HEALTHY

I remember someone saying to me, 'You don't see many fat vegetarians.'

But I've been vegetarian since I was nineteen, and yet that didn't mean I ate just vegetables and fruit. Being vegetarian or vegan doesn't automatically mean you're healthier than anyone else. You have to eat well, too. In fact, I became aneamic and had to introduce fish into my diet.

One of my vegan friends lives on veggie sausages, baguettes, chips and tomato pasta. And did you know Oreos and Ritz Crackers are vegan? I rest my case.

BOREDOM

Boredom = snacking. So keep busy!

TREATS & SNACKING

My treats don't come in a snack bag any more. A treat for me is no longer a KitKat or a big bag of salt and vinegar crisps. It's going to the M&S underwear department and being able to buy beautiful lingerie that I know I'll fit into. Or rewarding myself with some lovely flowers.

These days I just don't snack at all. My meals give me all the energy I need. But if you're desperate for something between meals, you can have a tiny handful of raisins, nuts or grapes. Be sensible.

PRIVATE PECKING

Just because no one can see you hiding behind the fridge door and eating cheese, it doesn't mean it's okay. Don't be an ostrich, sticking your head in the sand and telling yourself it's fine to cheat. It's not.

If you're hungry between meals, drink a pint of water with lemon or lime. Or have a herbal tea. People often mistake thirst for hunger.

Pecking equals pounds. You have to get yourself out of the habit.

SKIPPING MEALS

I've been guilty of this before, and you must not do it. You need to feed your body.

A TV can't turn on unless it's being fed electricity. You've got to keep your body ticking over, especially when you're exercising. It's like a sponge – and you'll be sweating so much, your sponge will dry out. You need to rehydrate it with food and water, and keep yourself going.

It's an utter travesty that people think they'll lose more weight by skipping meals. I don't get anywhere near as hungry now as I used to, so sometimes I'll set an alarm on my phone to remind myself to eat, because I would hate to skip lunch or dinner.

If you don't eat, your body goes into shock, switches into survival mode and holds on to any food you have had instead of burning it off. It's the 'Eskimo syndrome'. Fat will cling to you because your body thinks it needs it, and Eskimo fat is much harder to lose than normal fat.

You'll probably end up snacking and taking in more calories if you miss a meal, anyway. The best thing you can do is eat good, healthy meals with protein that will fill you up and give you lasting energy.

TELLING YOURSELF YOU'RE BIG-BONED

Have you ever seen a fat skeleton?

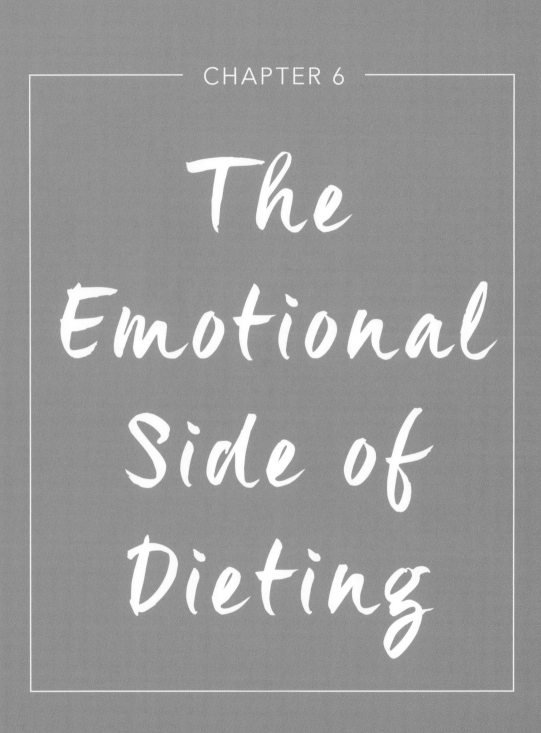

CHAPTER 6

The Emotional Side of Dieting

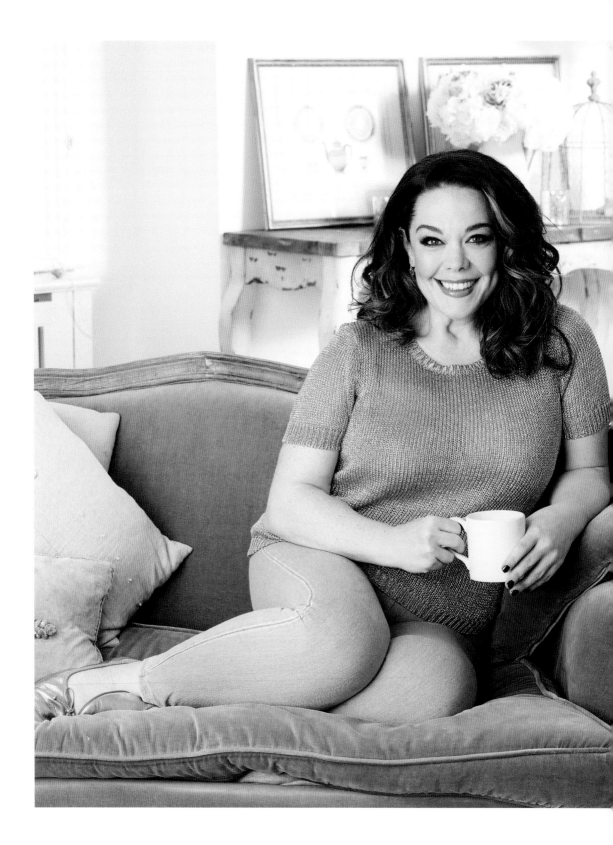

STUMBLING BLOCKS

Having been through all of this myself, I know dieting is about more than just what you eat. Emotions are a massive factor, and negative messages can have a huge impact.

So stop telling yourself *right now* that you can't lose weight. You can. Everyone can.

I know certain illnesses can make it slower or more difficult. But it doesn't mean it can't be done. If you tell yourself you can't lose weight, you won't. You have to believe you can.

Here are some of the main challenges that I came up against, and how to beat them.

NOT FEELING GOOD ENOUGH

I'm going to tell you something now and I want you to listen carefully:

YOU ARE GOOD ENOUGH AND YOU DESERVE TO FEEL AMAZING EVERY DAY.

Do you look at yourself in the mirror each day and tell yourself you're a failure because you can't lose weight? You're *not* a failure. Maybe it just wasn't the right time for you before. I was the same for a long time. Weight is a superficial thing. It's something you can – and will – change.

Stop seeing weight loss as a giant battle. Instead, see it as a series of small goals that will eventually add up and get you to where you want to be. Don't try to run before you can walk. Think of your journey as little lily pads you need to leap on to, one by one, to make your way across the pond.

Every tiny step forward is cause for celebration. But don't celebrate with an eclair! Food probably used to be your reward. You ate when you were up, when you were down, and probably at other times too. At first you may feel like you're taking that 'reward' away, and it needs to be replaced.

Exercising and seeing your body change week by week will become all the rewards you need, but on a very basic level it's important to celebrate each victory. Start an online wish list on your favourite shopping site. You can put anything on it – from a new pair of jeans to a gorgeous new Honesty Diary – but you must spoil yourself so that you don't look for rewards in the kitchen.Celebrate by giving yourself a massive pat on the back, and bask in that amazing feeling of achievement.

GIVING YOURSELF A HARD TIME

Imagine how much energy you've been using up giving yourself a hard time every day. From now on, put that energy into telling yourself how wonderful you are. Take it from me: the more weight you lose, the more you'll want to take care of your body because of how good you'll be feeling.

Every time you have one of those 'yay' moments, write it down in your Honesty Diary. If you feel this good already, just imagine how fantastic you're going to feel once you reach your overall goal:

Visualize how you're going to look.

Feel how you're going to feel.

Know what you're going to wear.

Make it real.

Think of me and know it's possible.

Believe you can do it, because YOU CAN!

Give yourself two minutes every morning when you wake up to appreciate how well you're doing, and carry that around with you all day.

Buy yourself an outfit you'd love to wear and hang it on the outside of your wardrobe so you see it every day. Imagine how incredible you're going to feel when you're wearing it. You need to bring that image of your new self to life.

I remember seeing a photo that someone took of my friends and me on a night out, when I was wearing an outfit I'd been dreaming of putting on for so long. I burst into tears when I saw it, because I wasn't the fat one any more. I realized that I blend in now. I look like other people.

I had nowhere to hide before, but now I can be anonymous. I can walk down the street and not be looked at. People may realize I'm 'Lisa off the telly', but they no longer stare at me because I'm fat.

I adore those moments. They help drive me on. You'll never get bored with feeling good. People always used to say to my mum, 'You must be so proud of Lisa.' Now I'm proud of myself.

DOING IT FOR THE WRONG REASONS

It's likely that part of the reason you want to lose weight is so you can be healthier and happier for your family. It may even be to impress your friends or your other half. But the bottom line is that the main reason you're losing weight has to be for you.

I worked with an amazing girl who tried everything to lose weight, including surgery. But she wasn't ever trying to lose weight for herself. She was doing it because all her friends were dating the cool lads, while she felt like the girl left on the bench at a prom, waiting for a guy to ask her to dance. She wanted to be slim so the cool boys would want to go out with her.

If you lose weight for a relationship and then you break up, what happens to your motivation?

The chances are you'll dive back into the biscuit tin.

This journey should be for you, first and foremost.

FEELING LIKE A BURDEN

Being on this diet does not make you a burden to other people. It may not always be easy for them if you're feeling down or you struggle sometimes, but you're much more of a burden while you're unhappy and overweight.

Do you want to face the possibility of getting type 2 diabetes? Or would you rather risk upsetting someone by taking your own food along to a get-together?

Would you rather people made comments about you being careful of what you eat? Or about you being overweight?

This is temporary! Friends and family aren't going to have to put up with the tricky moments forever, and neither are you. In fact, you're going to come out the other side happier, healthier and more positive than you've ever been.

THINKING YOU'RE SELFISH

When did it become selfish to want to be healthy?

Is it selfish to want to feel amazing and energized each day?

No! You are allowed to be your priority.

And it doesn't mean you love the people in your life any less. Successful people are usually the ones who value themselves. If you love yourself, you'll have more love to give out to others.

PLAYING A ROLE

Are you the fat, funny one? The bubbly, big person who's always laughing, even when you're feeling rubbish inside?

That was me.

Now?

I'm still funny, and I'm always laughing. But I'm no longer the butt of everyone's jokes. I'm still the girl I always was, but I'm a happier, more genuine version of me.

I stopped and thought to myself, 'Who am I? Who do I want to be?' That's when being me – the real me – became my priority.

For a long time I worried that my 'fat family' – the people who felt an affinity with me because I was big like them – would think I'd let them down and left them behind by losing weight. I felt guilty, as if I'd betrayed them. But I couldn't stay fat just to keep other people happy; we're all on our own journeys.

I've learned, more than ever, that you can't live your life for other people. And it turns out that they've all come along with me.

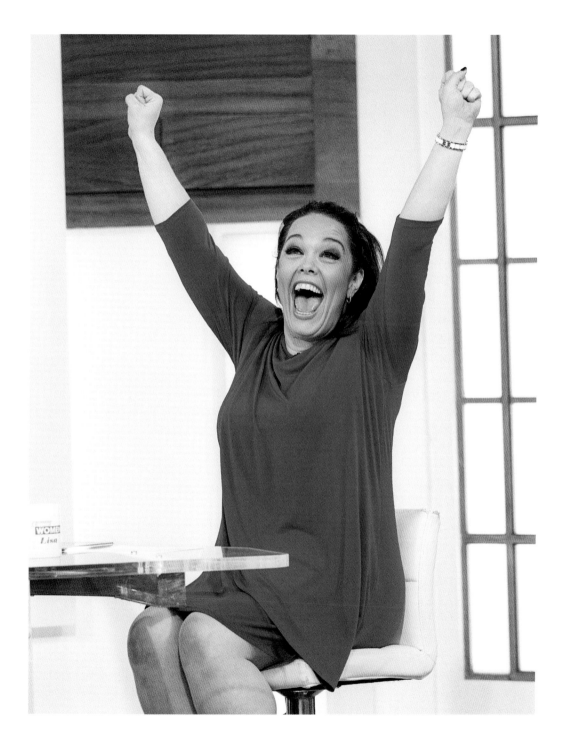

HIDING BEHIND YOUR FEARS

Is fear holding you back? Are you scared of losing the weight and still not feeling good enough?

Don't be. Take each day as it comes and write all these feelings down in your Honesty Diary. That's what it's there for.

The reality often turns out to be so much less scary than the thought of something.

FACING OTHER PEOPLE'S REACTIONS

This is such a tricky, sensitive subject but it needs addressing. Don't be surprised if your family and friends aren't always entirely supportive. They may not take you seriously at first.

How many times have you told them you're going on a diet? And how many times has it lasted just a day or two before they find you rummaging through the cupboards looking for crisps, or suggesting a cheeky takeaway?

They've seen you go to the gym and then come home and scoff fish and chips. It's likely their trust has gone. They've probably got diet disbelief after all this time. The words 'I really mean it this time' don't even register with them any more. They've stopped listening. So you've got to show them how serious you are.

Stop talking about it and do it!

When I first started this diet, I could almost hear my friends saying 'here we go again'. But the fact they didn't believe I would lose weight made me more determined than ever.

Let the doubters power you on.

Also be prepared that some people may be jealous of your progress, or paranoid that you're judging them, even when you're not.

I went for dinner with a friend recently and he didn't order dessert because he thought I'd be annoyed with him. As if! I don't care one bit what anyone else eats. I care what *I* eat. Just because I'm not eating cake, it doesn't mean I'm sitting up on a diet throne judging people who do.

One person's weight loss can shine a light on other people's extra pounds. If others in your family are big and you successfully slim down, suddenly they can't blame their genes any more.

When we used to go for a family meal, my dinner would be soup with a big wodge of bread, pasta with garlic bread, tiramisu for pudding, and a bottle of wine to myself. Now I'll have rocket and Parmesan for the starter, scallops for my main, and a coffee afterwards.

My family will say to me, 'You're not eating anything!'

But of course I am! I'm just not eating 3,000 calories in a single meal like I used to!

I worked with the gorgeous Abbey Clancy for a few months when I hosted the *Strictly* tour the year she took part in the show, and I was constantly taking the mickey out of her for eating nuts and seeds. I was always saying to her, 'Look at you nibbling on your rabbit food!'

Was it a defence mechanism, because she was tiny and I was obese? Yes. So when I hear others doing similarly, I know where it comes from.

Some of my friends and family have found it so hard getting used to me being smaller. They were used to 'Lisa the Leader'. I was large and in charge, and always the first one at the bar.

People in your life may fear you changing, because they don't know how to handle it. Change can be terrifying for some people.

When I first went out for meals with friends and ordered a salad while they ate pizza, they'd say, 'Are you okay?' Really they were saying, 'I'm not sure if I'm okay with this.'

Another thing people said to me a lot was, 'Don't lose any more weight or you won't be you.'

But I'm still me! I've lost 12 stone and had some flabby skin cut off but I'm still Lisa, inside and out. I'm still opinionated and I still find the same things funny. I didn't lose my personality along with the weight.

I've still got the same friends I've always had. None of them went running for the hills because I'm half the size I once was. It just took a little bit of time for them to get used to the new me. And now they're just happy that I'm happy.

People will soon get used to the new, improved you.

BEING SCARED OF COMPLIMENTS

Even now I struggle to accept compliments, because they take me back to the time when my skin was saggy, before my surgery.

People would tell me how wonderful I looked and all I could think was, 'You have no idea what I look like under these clothes.' It was like I'd let the helium out of a giant balloon. I'd worked so hard, but I still didn't feel worthy. In response, I wanted to say to everyone, 'Thanks so much for being nice but I'm really not finished yet.'

Sometimes compliments come in funny guises. I was food shopping a while ago. I put my items on the conveyor belt and then two grannies got in the queue behind me. They kept looking over so I smiled and one of them said, 'Sorry for staring. It's just that we thought you were Lisa Riley, but she's miles fatter than you.'

I laughed so much I thought I was going to wet myself. It was such a brilliant moment.

Nowadays, if someone says something nice to me – even if I'm not having the most confident of days – I'll say thank you and accept it.

Please, please, please do the same. Drink up every nice thing that's said to you.

It may take a bit of practice, but you'll soon get the hang of it. Set aside some blank pages in your Honesty Diary (you're going to need quite a few). Write down every time someone gives you a compliment, and reread them often.

People give us compliments to make us feel good about ourselves, so let's use them for precisely that.

LET'S FEEL AMAZING! IT'S YOUR DIVINE RIGHT!

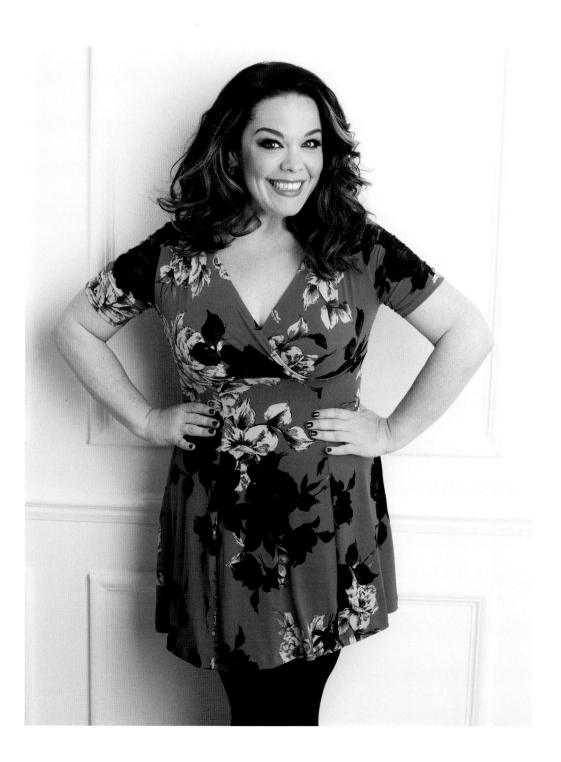

CHAPTER 7

My Food Rules

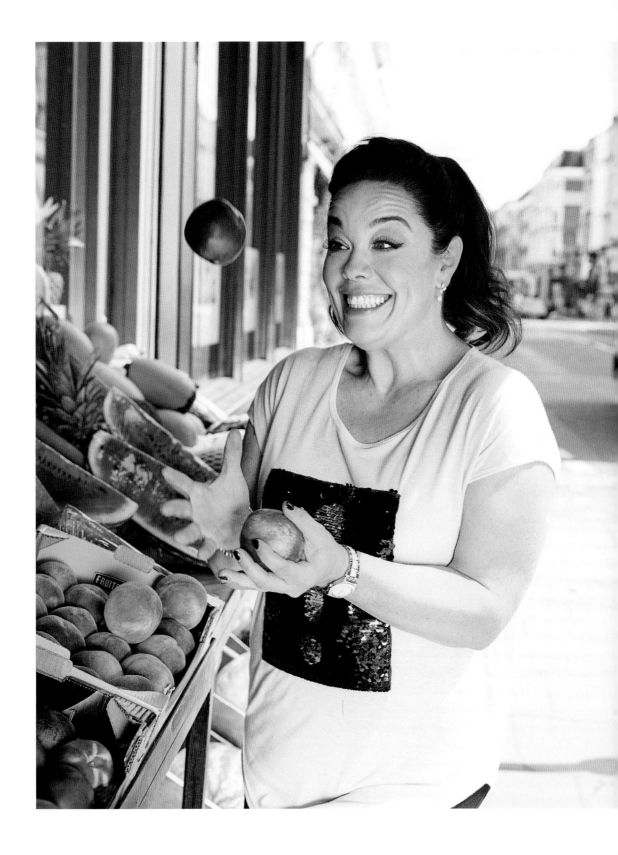

These are the food rules I learned to stick to on my diet. Even now I'm slimmer, I still try to follow them as closely as I can. If you can introduce all or most of these habits into your diet, you should see a big difference.

SAY GOODBYE TO WHITE CARBS

I recommend having no potatoes, rice, pasta or bread on this diet until later on down the line, once you've done the initial hard work and you're maintaining a reduced weight. And, even then, be cautious, go for brown or wholegrain varieties, and certainly don't have them every day.

I didn't eat any kind of white carbs for a long time when I started dieting, and even now I'm very careful with them. I'll have them sometimes, but they're not a regular thing for me.

Bread is everywhere and really hard to avoid. One really helpful tip: if you go out to eat at a restaurant, ask them not to bring bread so you're not tempted. You can easily end up eating a basketful before you've even ordered. And don't think that a sandwich is the only option for lunch. Have a healthy soup or salad instead.

Can you do without potatoes on your plate? Yes, you can. There is no rule that you must have potatoes, bread or pasta with dinner. So don't! If you feel like your meal looks too small without them, the answer is to add lots more lovely fresh vegetables. The more veg in your diet, the better!

AVOID SUGAR

You will have sugar cravings at times, but they're temporary and they will go. If I have a sweet craving I'll have some fruit.

People say to me, 'But there's sugar in fruit.'

And yes, there is – but it's natural. Fructose (the sugar found in fruit) is encased in fibre, which helps the body absorb it more slowly, so we don't get a big, sudden sugar hit. Whereas added sugars metabolize very quickly, causing a sugar spike and then a crash back down, which often makes you crave even more sugar. Added sugar has a lot of calories and zero health benefits.

A small handful of chilled seedless grapes will take away sugar cravings instantly. I swear to God it works (take it from me, I've tried everything).

If you must have sugar in tea and coffee, I would actually recommend sugar instead of sweeteners – which I hate, because they're so artificial. Ideally, you'll stop having sugar in hot drinks, but you don't have to go cold turkey. Wean yourself off, a little bit at a time. Start by cutting out a quarter of your portion, and keep reducing until you're just having a smidgen in every cup. Then eventually you'll be able to cut it out completely.

Please don't ever use sugar substitutes. Keep it real. Have you noticed that you don't get substitutes for real food – like fruit and vegetables? That's because you don't need them. Because the real deal is so good for you.

If you shouldn't be having sugar, you certainly shouldn't be having an unnatural substitute. These days, I keep a tub of cinnamon in my kitchen to naturally sweeten foods. You can even add it to your coffee!

DITCH THE DIET DRINKS

STAY AWAY! These are not the dieter's friend. Just like what happens with added sugars, the fake saccharin in diet drinks will, in fact, make you crave more sugar.

The only drinks I have now are coffee, tea (regular and herbal), and still and sparkling water. I occasionally have cranberry juice as a treat or if I'm out with my friends, and I'll have a skinny mocha when I've got bad PMT!

MILK IT

Not to get all clean eating here, but personally I prefer unsweetened almond milk to cow's milk, these days. I used to have a pint of whole milk as a drink, which horrifies me now. I can't be one hundred per cent certain, but I suspect lactose caused water retention for me, which can happen to some people, and I do feel better now I don't have it. If you think you might have an intolerance, it's worth getting tested. Your GP can advise on this. Otherwise, there's no reason to cut out milk, as it contains protein and calcium, which your body needs. Just make sure to drink it in moderation and ideally stick to the red tops (skimmed) if you like the real stuff, as it has fewer calories.

A LITTLE BIT CHEESY

People may find it surprising that I include some cheese on my diet, but allow me to explain! I eat halloumi and Parmesan because they're incredibly flavoursome. A little goes a long way, and they're full of protein.

Halloumi is so rich, it's hard to have more than three or four squares. And you only need a small bit of Parmesan to give something a really good kick. It's all about getting flavour into your food.

I avoid those pre-grated grab bags of cheddar at all costs. They contain such a huge amount – if you were to equate how much is in them to a block of cheese, you would be shocked. Someone actually said to me that they think grated cheese is okay because it's mostly air. It tricks your mind, and you end up eating loads more than you would otherwise.

People think pizzas aren't that bad, because they look like they don't have much cheese on them. But if you were to scoop up all the cheese and form it back into a block, you'd be horrified by how much you're consuming. It's like one of those optical illusions; it deceives you.

NO 'PING' MEALS

I ate a lot of ready meals back in the day. I was very guilty of the 'single ping'. I can't even begin to imagine how many tuna pasta bakes I put in the microwave.

The day McCain brought out Micro Chips will forever be etched on my mind. I was euphoric. I could have a box of chips straight from the microwave, and I ate them like there was no tomorrow. Not only that, I'd also have a packet of crisps while I was waiting for them to cook.

'Ping meals' are full of crap, so a lot of them can block you up. And the diet ones are often the worst for that. You're being sold a convenience dream, but I'm afraid they're not going to make you lose weight – even if they claim they will. It's not about the calorie count: it's about all the rubbish they contain.

DON'T TAP THE APP

It's so easy to eat badly these days. You can order a pizza on an app on your way home and it will be waiting for you when you get to your door.

No wonder we're all overweight!

From now on, takeaways won't be a part of your life. Even if you go for the 'healthy' options, you don't know what's in them. The only way you'll know is by cooking your own food. Read on . . . !

ADIOS MEAL DEALS

Step away from the meal deal. There was a time when people would just have a sandwich for lunch. Now it's often cheaper to buy a deal with crisps, a sugary drink and maybe even a dessert thrown in. Sandwiches and crisps have become as thick as thieves and we've been taught they go hand in hand.

You tell yourself you won't eat the lot. But, let's face it, we all do.

And if you go for a fast-food meal you are presented with deals where you can get a huge portion for just a little more money.

So why wouldn't you 'go large'? Because you're going to gain pounds for those extra pennies, that's why.

All-you-can-eat buffets and carveries didn't exist when I was growing up, but now they're everywhere. Everyone wants their money's worth, these days. So we've ended up eating tons more than we actually need.

I think you know what I'm going to say: no meal deals, all-you-can-eats or carveries while you're on this diet.

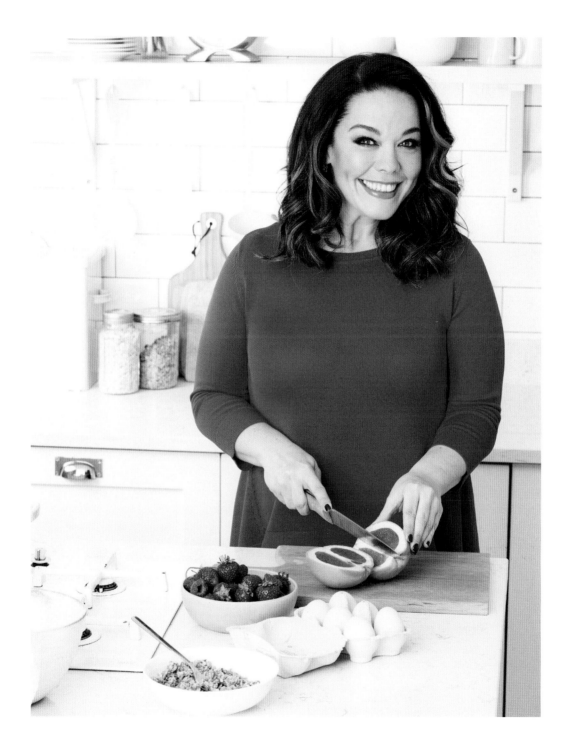

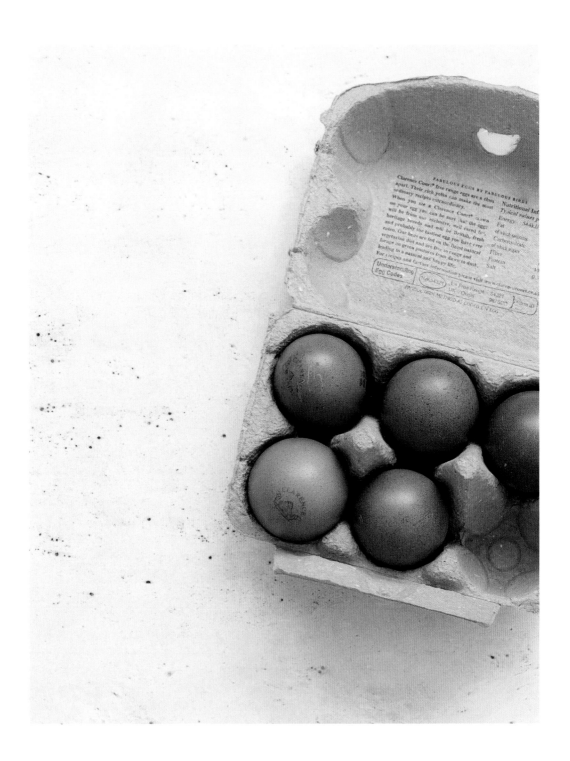

DEEP-FRIED = FAT

Deep-frying is the most unhealthy way of cooking something.

Some people think that if they have sweet potato fries with a meal, they're being good. But the clue is in the name – fries!

They may be slightly healthier than normal chips but they're still packed with fat from the oil they've been fried in.

DUMP THE DIET FOODS

Anything that has to tell you how good it is for you on the packet probably isn't. Most diet foods are a myth and contain just as many calories as the everyday ones. You're so much better off having a banana than a packet of 'low fat' crisps.

Some of the best advice I can give you is to always think 'fresh'. That doesn't mean you have to go to a posh farmers' market every Saturday and spend a fortune on organic produce. But do try to eat as naturally as possible.

Please don't think it's going to be more expensive to eat fresh food either, because it's really not. Lidl's and Aldi's amazing fruit and veg aisles are very reasonable, as are greengrocers and local markets. You can get such great bargains! You'll find loads of ideas for how to use fresh produce in the recipe section (see pages 139–251).

EGGS ARE YOUR BEST FRIENDS

Eggs can be eaten in so many different ways, and they're amazing for filling you up.

Packed with protein, incredibly versatile and always cheap, these little buddies appear a lot in my recipes.

SPICE UP YOUR LIFE

If your food isn't varied, you'll soon get bored and slip into old ways. Livening up all your food with spices is an easy way to keep it interesting.

Try new things, even if you don't know if you'll like them. I always thought I hated coriander, and now it's one of the things I use most in dishes to give them a great flavour kick.

You need to be tickling your taste buds at all times.

COOK FROM SCRATCH

I know it's not always possible. But if you cook from scratch, you'll always be in control of what you put in your mouth. And you'll be able to be totally honest with yourself about what you've eaten.

Don't waste your time reading the back of packets for calories when you could be spending that time cooking real food. Use your common sense. You know a creamy, cheese-laden pasta dish isn't going to be good for you.

If you pay attention to your food, eating well will soon become second nature to you. You'll quickly learn which healthy ingredients you love to eat and how to make delicious dishes with them.

COOK IN BATCHES

Batch cooking is a total game changer. If you're making a big chilli, make double and freeze half.

It will mean you'll have quick, healthy meals in the house when you need them, and you won't be tempted to cheat.

Embrace your freezer. This is where your old takeaway containers are going to come in handy! Some of my food rules – such as not eating too late – are much easier to stick to if you've got healthy food in the freezer, ready to reheat, so that you don't have to rush in from work and cook a whole meal from scratch.

BRANCH OUT

I used to be terrified of anything that was 'good' for me. I didn't ever choose the healthy option. I didn't really understand the appeal of things like lentils and chickpeas, so they didn't even register with me.

As for recipes, I always thought, 'Why make something when I can buy it? That's what shops are for, surely?' I never, ever thought, 'I can't wait to get home and make a lovely king prawn and coriander salad.' I wanted to buy one already made up in a plastic bowl.

Now, I love creating my own meals. It's not just healthier, but also rewarding.

I feel a real sense of achievement when I cook a meal from scratch – and you will, too.

WATCH YOUR PORTIONS

I cannot say this enough:

YOUR PORTIONS NEED TO BE SMALLER IF YOU WANT TO LOSE WEIGHT!

If your stomach is used to being fed big portions, it now needs to get used to having smaller ones. Your stomach is in training. And, honestly, once you're used to it, you'll wonder how you ever ate as much as you used to.

BOWLS ARE BEST

I deliberately don't have any plates in my house. I always use a bowl, because they're so much harder to overfill.

Swap your plate for a bowl. It's a simple method of portion control that really works.

STOP WHEN YOU'RE FULL

This is a really hard one, and it took me a while to retrain my body and mind to know when I was full. Quite often people who have spent years yo-yo dieting have lost the ability to stop when they're full, because they're locked in a feast-or-famine cycle. They're either hugely restricting what they eat and only eating 'diet' foods, or they're off a diet and eating everything they can get their hands on.

It's about finding that middle ground, which takes practice.

Eat slowly and mindfully, by putting your fork down between mouthfuls to let your brain keep up with your belly. If you do this often enough, it will soon become a permanent habit.

As soon as you've finished eating, move your bowl out of sight. If there is any food left, it could end up tempting you. You could find yourself doing some 'why not?' picking.

ALWAYS SIT DOWN TO EAT

Be mindful every time you eat. Sit down and make sure you don't have anything to distract you. Give the food all your attention. Eat slowly and chew well. You have spent time making this delicious food, so you should enjoy every mouthful.

SHOP SMALLER

I know this isn't always possible if you've got a family, a demanding job and a busy schedule, but I stopped doing a weekly bulk shop and started doing a couple of smaller shops instead. When I did one big shop, I'd often end up panic-buying extra items. It was like I'd forgotten the shops were open every day. We've all been guilty of buying food we don't need. And it meant my fridge would be crammed full of too many temptations.

If you genuinely don't have time to visit the shops more than once a week, as I know many people don't when they're juggling work and families, you just need to be really careful and disciplined about what you buy. Make a list before you go and stick to it.

My top tip is to eat something before you do a supermarket shop. It's shocking how much more food you'll want to put in your basket if you're hungry.

Also beware of the 'deals' in supermarkets. Just because you're saving 2p on an extra packet of biscuits, it doesn't mean you should buy them. And, let's be honest, if they're in the cupboard you'll end up eating them.

DON'T HAVE TEMPTING FOOD IN THE HOUSE

Don't buy food 'just in case' you fancy it. Because then you probably will fancy it.

When I was giving up smoking, I'd keep a pack of ten cigarettes 'just in case'. And guess what? I kept smoking them. It's too easy.

Don't have naughty foods stashed in the cupboards. If you went to a shop and they didn't have what you wanted in stock, then you wouldn't be able to buy it. It's the same at home – if you don't have sweets and crisps 'in stock', then you can't eat them. Your partner and/or children may complain about this, but think about the great example you'll be setting for them, too! If they really can't cope without, perhaps you could ask your partner or a friend to shop for those items, and then insist they are hidden somewhere you don't know about and won't be able to find!

HAVE YOUR OWN CUPBOARD

If you share your kitchen with family, friends or flatmates, having your own kitchen cupboard is essential. Empty out an entire cupboard and fill it with the foods you're going to need while you're on this plan (see my recommendations on page 141). Make everyone aware that it's your cupboard, and they're not allowed to put anything extra in it. Likewise, don't look in their cupboards unless you're cooking for them.

Remove anything that may tempt you. I hate throwing food away, so I either gave it to mates, or I put things like raspberry jam way out of my reach so I couldn't see them and be tempted to pick at them. Get your family to hide things if need be.

USE YOUR FOOD

I don't like seeing food go to waste. Eating healthily on my diet plan has the added bonus that you will be using lots of lovely fresh ingredients. If anything is going out of date, and you really don't think it will last, then cook or freeze it. If you've got leftover fresh fruit and vegetables, put them in your blender and make a smoothie, or freeze them for another time, or add them to the frittata or omelette muffin recipes you'll find on pages 194 and 196. It's a great way of getting good nutrients into your system while also saving a few pennies.

Use your common sense. Yes, things have sell-by dates, but you can see and smell whether food is still okay to eat. A brown banana isn't going to kill you.

STICK TO WHAT YOU LIKE

Dieting shouldn't be a torturous process. There are so many nice things you can enjoy, so why eat foods you don't like? If you're not a fan of cucumber, don't eat it! Simple as that.

The word 'diet' no longer means boring, bland food. We're not living in the 1970s and existing on three grapefruits a day in order to drop pounds. There are so many more choices, these days.

JAZZ UP SALADS

Salad does not have to be rabbit food. Keep your salads chunky by adding chickpeas, butter beans, tomatoes, roasted vegetables – anything fresh and healthy goes. These foods are great for your digestion, so you might feel a bit windy afterwards. But your body will love you!

However, be aware that putting something in a salad bowl doesn't make it a salad. Potatoes and mayonnaise are two dieting no-nos. Just because you can combine them and call it a 'potato salad' does not mean it's healthy. Some shops sell tubs of pasta, tuna and mayonnaise mixed together and labelled as a salad. If you picked apart the ingredients, the only salad in there is probably a little bit of sweetcorn and maybe some grated carrot at the bottom.

Don't trust everything that has 'salad' written on it.

Oh, and absolutely no croutons! They're packed with fat and calories.

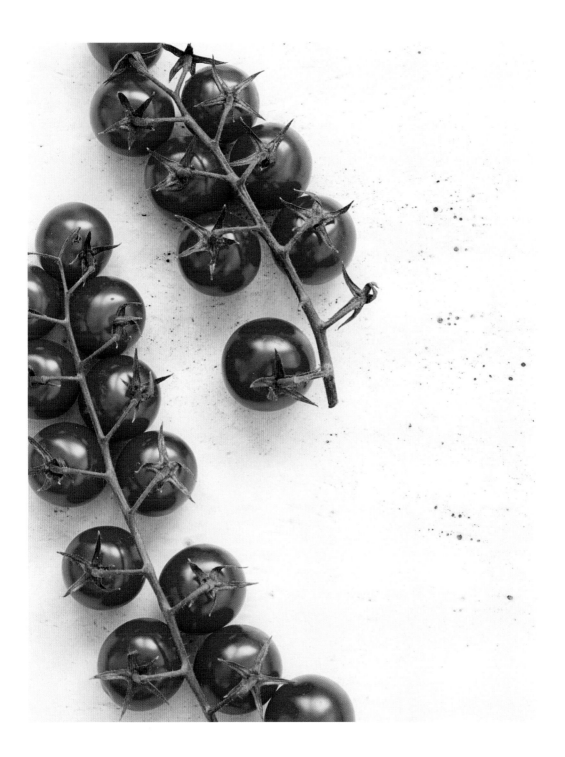

DON'T EAT LATE

I know this one is hard, but I find it makes a real difference. It gives your body and digestive system a chance to have a rest and properly process the food you've eaten during the day. The following morning, you'll be hungry for a good breakfast and your body will be ready to burn it efficiently.

My personal cut-off time is 6.30 p.m., but I know everyone's lives are different and if you work long hours you might be worrying about how to get home in time to make this happen. But if you eat your main meal at lunchtime, then your evening food can be kept very quick and simple to put together. Preparing things in advance can also help, meaning you can pull healthy homemade food out of the fridge or freezer and it's ready to eat fast. It doesn't have to be an exact science, but it is best to eat a few hours before you go to bed, not least because it can disrupt your sleep. Aim to eat before you settle down to watch *Corrie* or *EastEnders*!

If you know you won't be back home till late, perhaps take food with you in a lunchbox or thermos to make sure you don't miss dinner. It takes a bit of planning and I know there will be times when life gets in the way, but it's worth trying to stick to this rule whenever you realistically can.

BUTTER OVER MARGARINE

I'd prefer you not to have either. But if you *have* to use one or the other every now and again, please always go for the butter because it's the more natural of the two.

WATER IS KEY

If you get hungry, drink water. A lot of it. If you find water boring, add flavour by squeezing a lemon, lime or orange into it, or have herbal tea instead. Your body often mistakes thirst for hunger, so drink to shrink! It works.

GET YOUR FAMILY TO HELP

If you're making spaghetti Bolognese and garlic bread for your family, it's going to tempt all your senses and make you hungry. Will you be able to resist it? If you don't think you can, then you could ask your partner, friend or a family member to make dinner for the rest of the household for a couple of weeks until you're well into your dieting stride (though I'm aware this won't be a realistic option for everyone!). Let them know it won't be forever, but it's especially important in the beginning, when you need as much help as possible. If you're a single parent, or your partner isn't keen on cooking, make sure you eat your own dinner before you start cooking for others, so you're not tempted to do any picking.

PICKERS WEAR BIG KNICKERS!

Making two separate meals may feel time consuming, but this is a huge investment. Again, it can help to keep healthy meals pre-prepared in the fridge or freezer so that your own food is quick to pull out and you don't end up spending your entire evening cooking.

I'm not saying mealtimes will be easy. It may be difficult watching your family tuck into shepherd's pie while you're having soup. And if your kids tend not to finish their meals, please don't pick at leftovers from their plates. (I hate waste, so if there's any food that's worth saving pop it in the fridge – out of sight! – and you can give it to the kids the following day.)

If you find it too hard, why not take yourself away while your family or partner is eating? You could go to the gym or for a walk, have a nice long bath, or watch your favourite TV show? Reward yourself and remove yourself from the dinner table so you don't feel like you're missing out.

BE CLEVER

Tweak healthy recipes so your family can also enjoy them. If you're making yourself a healthy curry, there's no reason why your family can't enjoy it, too. They needn't know how virtuous it is! Add popadoms, naans or chapattis to theirs, if need be. Don't you dare take one for yourself, though!

TAKE LUNCH WITH YOU

If you're often away from home at lunchtime, it's a good idea to take lunch with you, if practical. It needn't take long to prepare a healthy lunch the night before, and you'll be less likely to grab unhealthy convenience food if you've brought food with you. Invest in a lunchbox or thermos flask (for soup), and don't forget that it's best to eat your bigger meal at lunchtime. If your workplace has a fridge and a microwave, you definitely have no excuse not to have a good lunch! And if you find yourself out and about at lunchtime, resist the temptation to just grab a sandwich, easy as that can be. Even the simplest cafés usually serve soup or omelettes, and there are so many delicious (healthy!) salads available from supermarkets and coffee shops.

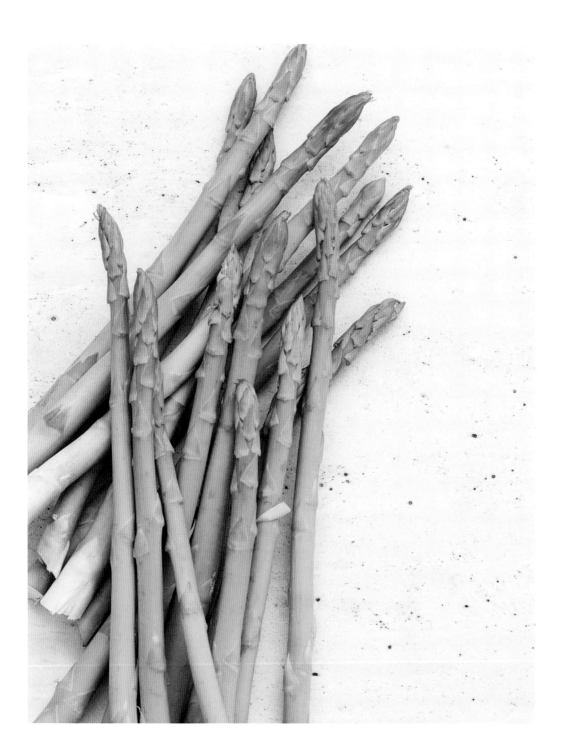

BE WISE WHEN YOU DINE

Ideally, you won't be eating out too regularly while you're doing this plan. But if you do, you want to be able to enjoy yourself without ruining your diet. (If you don't think you can trust yourself to stick to your diet, I'm sorry to say it, but it's best you don't go at all.)

I would recommend ordering two healthy starters, rather than one big main. Soup and prawns are good options. Garlic pizza bread is not!

A lot of restaurant chains put nutritional information online now, so you can always check out some good options before you leave the house.

Don't be afraid to ask the waiter or waitress about the healthiest menu options, and tell them if you want your chicken grilled instead of fried and your salad dressing served on the side.

Be sensible about where you eat out. If you were a vegetarian, you wouldn't go to a steak house. So why would you go for a greasy Chinese or heavy Indian when you're on a diet? Use your common sense when choosing where to dine. Italian restaurants are by far the best places to go, because they do great salads, meat and fish.

If you're going to someone's house for dinner, this is a place where honesty comes in. If you don't know the hosts very well, it could potentially be awkward if you shoo away the dessert, so let them know upfront you're on a serious diet. If you know someone really, really well, and you know they won't mind you taking your own food along with you, do it. Barbecues are a real diet win. Okay, so you can't have the buns and coleslaw, but prawn kebabs, low-fat barbecued meat and salads are all great. If contributions are welcome, take healthy options along with you to make sure there's something suitable for you to eat.

If you're off to a party and worried about losing control and wolfing down canapés or cake, eat before you go, or take healthy snacks in your bag. Parents are so good at making sure they've got everything their kids need when they're out, so why not do the same for yourself?

HONESTY ALL THE WAY!

Finally, ask yourself every day – how honest are you really being? If you think you're veering off track, pull yourself back. You've got all the tools now, so there are no excuses!

CHAPTER 8

Your Life-Changing, 8-Day Kick-Start

It's Week 1! This is when things are going to start to turn around for you.

ARE YOU EXCITED? YOU SHOULD BE!

When it comes to this diet, I'm not going to try and baffle you with loads of different stages where you have to cut out foods before reintroducing them.

I want it to be as simple as it can be.

But I will say that the first thing you need to do is show your body you mean business, and that means cutting your food intake right down by following my 8-Day Kick-Start plan.

I went to a weight-loss boot camp when I very first started out, and it was integral to changing my thought patterns and showing me what my body was capable of. It proved to me that I'd been lying to myself all this time and that I was capable of losing weight, after all. But it wasn't going to be a walk in the park.

For years, I'd told myself that one day the pounds might magically start to fall off and my body would find its natural weight. If you've been thinking the same, here's a newsflash – it just ain't going to happen!

Unless you change your thinking and eating long term, you'll always be overweight.

This kick-start plan is about saying to your body, 'Can you hear me, loud and clear? I don't want to be overweight any more.' It's designed to produce rapid weight loss initially. I won't pretend it's easy, but seeing a big difference after eight days will give you a great confidence boost and lots of motivation to keep going.

And, as the Russian dancers used to tell me on *Strictly*, if it doesn't hurt, you're not doing it properly.

You're effectively stripping your body of nasty old wallpaper before you redecorate. But first you have to get right down to the bare plaster, so your body can be thoroughly revamped.

It's going to take time and energy, but it will be so worth it.

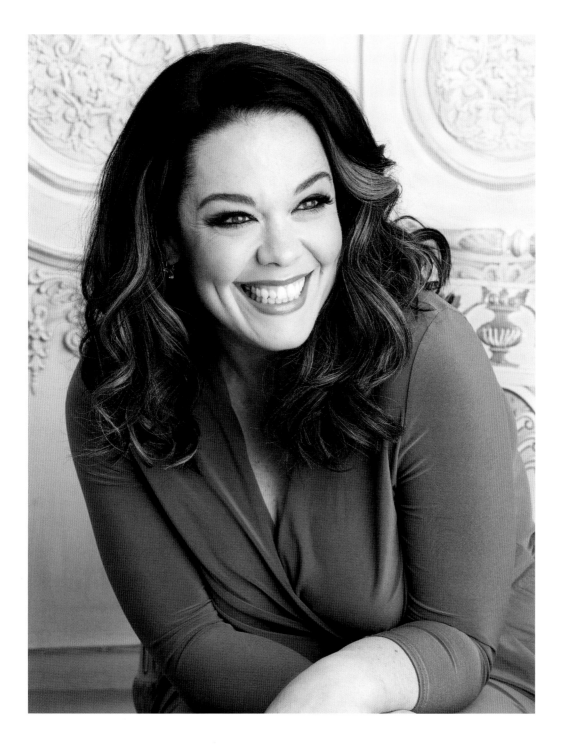

Before you run for the hills, consider this – it's only eight days out of the tens of thousands you'll live in your life. Eight days. Not much more than a week. In the grand scheme of things, it's nothing!

We all know the saying – if at first you don't succeed, give yourself a kick up the backside and try again. If you do fall off the wagon, pick yourself up and give it another go.

There is no limit to how many times you can take that first step. The most important thing is that you take it.

I actually followed an even stricter diet than this when I went to the weight-loss boot camp. It's widely known that it involved only 400–500 calories a day. But I wasn't trying to go about my usual daily life at the same time – yes, I had to do lots of exercise, but I was also able to get plenty of sleep and rest, and I wasn't at work during that week. It was also supervised by professionals. I know that most people doing my plan will be unsupervised and trying to fit the diet into their everyday life, so for this book I've developed a slightly more forgiving plan, still designed to get quick results, but which most people should be able to follow safely, no matter your starting point.

During the Kick-Start, you may get hungry and feel a bit rubbish at times, as your body adjusts to receiving less food. Drink a lot of water to help stay hydrated. If you currently drink a lot of tea and coffee, you may also experience caffeine withdrawal, often in the form of headaches, but you can get through this. Cutting down gradually can help avoid symptoms. If you really do drink a lot of caffeine, it's actually a good idea to start cutting down in advance, otherwise you'll find yourself suffering the effects of cold turkey while also trying to start your diet – which won't put you in the best frame of mind for success. Try switching to decaf, herbal tea or hot water with lemon, so that you can still enjoy hot drinks but without the caffeine.

If processed food has been your drug for a long time, your body is going to be surprised when you take that away, and there's inevitably going to be a period of readjustment there too.

You need to start as you mean to go on. Just think how amazing you're going to feel afterwards.

It's really important to be as kind to yourself as you can during this time. Your portions will be small and your exercise level will be high, so try to get as much sleep as possible so your body has a chance to recover, heal and re-energize. You'll need to rest your body ready for the following day.

This first week is going to be tough, but it's when you're going to start losing weight and your body start burning fat. You'll consume minimal calories, carbs and fat – much less than you're used to. You'll often have your main meal at lunchtime, and ideally you'll eat less in the evening so your body has a decent amount of time to do some serious fat burning overnight.

After the initial 8-Day Kick-Start, it's time to ease your body into your new long-term eating regime. Once you've finished the plan you can embark on your new life-long eating routine by following my food rules, as I outlined in Chapter 7.

As for exercise, you need to sweat every single day while on the plan, and ideally afterwards too. I'm very strict about that. You need to be doing different cardio, and mixing it up. And if your clothes aren't wet, you haven't worked out properly. You need to be working your body to the max, because that's when you start to see big changes.

There's a difference between doing exercise to be healthy, doing exercise to become toned and doing exercise to burn fat. At this stage you want to be burning fat, and that means at least forty-five minutes of cardio a day. That may sound like a lot. If you haven't exercised for some time, you might need to take things slowly to start with and build up, which is fine, too. Start small and build up by five minutes a day until you get up to the full forty-five minutes.

We'll talk more about exercise later in the book, so please do read Chapter 9 'Move It!' before you start.

One thing I should mention is that you usually go to the toilet more when you start a diet and your body begins working as it should. Don't be too posh to talk about poo. Everyone does it, and you should be doing it more than ever on this plan.

Listen to your body. If you're visiting the loo a lot it's such a good thing, because it means your body is ticking over well and processing your food efficiently. Ideally, you want to poo an hour or two after every meal you eat, and at the very least once a day. If you think you're not pooing enough, have an apple or a handful of berries to help move things along.

THE 8-DAY KICK-START

IMPORTANT

Before you start, it's very important for me to say that this diet is not suitable for pregnant or breastfeeding women, nor for children, teenagers, those with a history of eating disorders or anyone who is frail or unwell. You should consult with your doctor or a healthcare professional before embarking on the plan, to ensure you are in good health and to make sure it's the right choice for you, especially if you are on any kind of medication or treatment plan. It's always a good idea to get medical advice, particularly if you have a lot of weight to lose, in which case I also recommend you seek the guidance of a registered nutritionist if you can.

HELPFUL TIPS

Once you're ready, here are a few handy tips to make sure you get off to a great start.

- You'll begin each day with hot water and lemon (either fresh or bottled, and as much as you like), which will help to invigorate and rehydrate you. The vitamin C in the lemon will also give your immune system a little boost.

- Drink loads of water. At least two litres a day, and more if you can. Water is your ally. It will help stop you feeling hungry. The same part of your brain deals with hunger and thirst signals, so it can be easy to confuse them. Sometimes when you think you're hungry, you may just need a big glass of water.

- Feel free to drizzle salad and vegetables with a little balsamic vinegar and salt and pepper to season and liven them up!

- If you decide to swap in or add extra vegetables, make sure it's not potatoes of any kind!

- If there's anything on the plan you really don't like, or can't eat for some reason or because you're vegetarian, you can of course replace it with a meal from another day or another recipe from the book with a roughly similar number of calories (though please steer clear of the sweet potato and couscous recipes while on the initial plan). It's fine to mix and match a little bit.

- Please remember there should be no snacking between meals, or the plan won't work effectively. If you're absolutely desperate, a few almonds or grapes will help you through, but try your absolute hardest to resist. And I do MEAN just a few.

	BREAKFAST	LUNCH	DINNER
DAY 1	Hot water and lemon Scrambled eggs with chive, spring onion and avocado (p.148)	Sesame steak stir-fry (p.202)	Spicy carrot and lentil soup (p.184) (make enough for two days)
DAY 2	Hot water and lemon Pimped-up yoghurt (p.153)	Spicy carrot and lentil soup (leftover portion from previous day)	Tuna and bean salad (p.167)
DAY 3	Hot water and lemon Bury berry smoothie (p.146)	Lentil, feta and tomato salad (p168)	Garlic and chilli cod with roasted spinach and cauliflower (p.226)
DAY 4	Hot water and lemon Strictly healthy porridge (p.144)	Simple tomato soup (p.178) (make enough for two days)	Chicken and asparagus tray bake (p.206)
DAY 5	Hot water and lemon Granola with fresh raspberries (p.149) and low-fat natural yoghurt	Simple tomato soup (leftover portion from previous day)	Grilled salmon with basil, garlic and wilted spinach (p.208)
DAY 6	Hot water and lemon Bury berry smoothie (p.146)	Vegetable frittata (p.194) with a mixed salad	Sesame prawn salad (p.174)
DAY 7	Hot water and lemon Scrambled eggs with chive, spring onion and avocado (p.148)	Chunky chicken and vegetable broth (p.179) (make enough for two days)	Baked aubergine with tomato and halloumi (p.223)
DAY 8	Hot water and lemon Strictly healthy porridge (p.144)	Chunky chicken and vegetable broth (leftover portion from previous day)	Lemon prawns (p.213)

DON'T FORGET TO CELEBRATE!

After these eight days you should really begin to notice differences in your body, your skin and your energy levels.

CONGRATULATIONS!

Make sure you note down all of these changes and achievements in your Honesty Diary. Now is also a great time to look back at the questionnaire you answered at the start of this book (see pages 15–17). Have any of your answers changed? I bet some have, particularly about the way you eat. Jot down any updates or new answers.

This is all brilliant, but, whatever you do, don't celebrate your weight loss with food or booze!

Buy yourself a nice treat instead – maybe some new workout gear, pretty flowers or an indulgent candle or bath essence. This is all about you taking care of yourself in the best way possible, without using chocolate or wine as a reward. Each time you buy yourself something lovely, remind yourself how well you're doing and how much you're worth it.

So what next? Well, if you feel able and ready to, you're more than welcome to follow the plan again! You could wait a few days, or you can do it back to back. It depends how hard you found it and how you feel now. Otherwise, it's time to start using my food rules (see page 89) and all my other healthy recipes that I've included in the book. You can follow the 8-Day Kick-Start again at any point in the future, whenever you're in need of some fast progress or a bit of a boost.

This is it now! This is how things are going to be for the rest of your life. You are going to wake up feeling proud of yourself every single day. You're never going back to the old you – and the new you deserves to be spoilt and feel incredible!

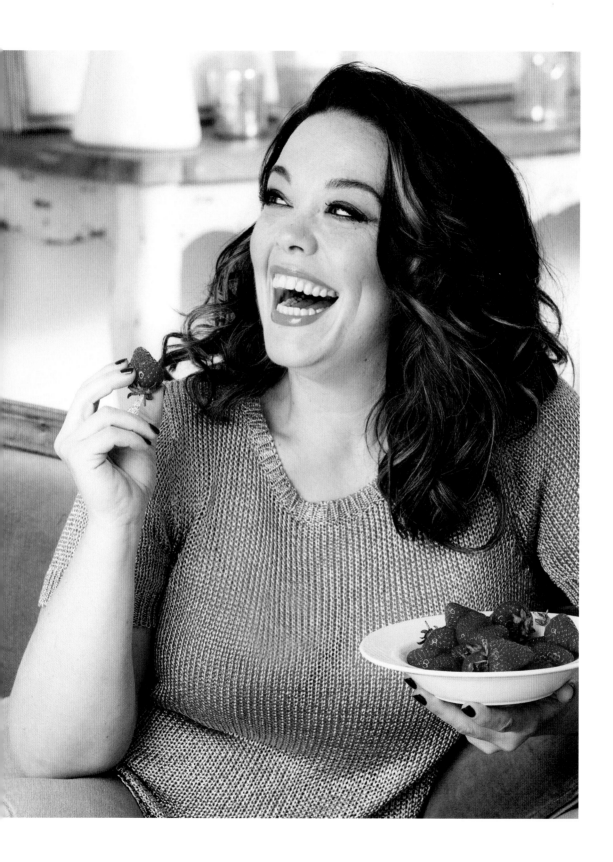

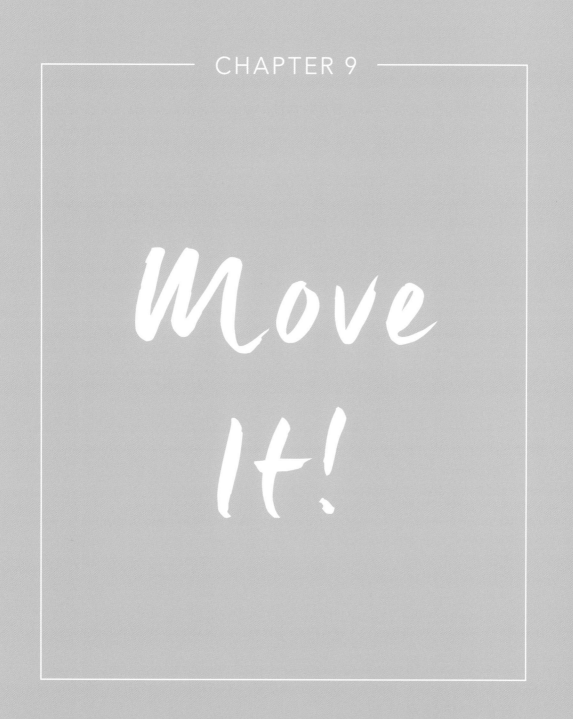

CHAPTER 9

Move It!

WEIGHT LOSS COSTS

Here's where you start paying – in sweat!

I guess I had a bit of a head start when it came to getting into exercise because the training I did with *Strictly* taught me that I could do it, in spite of my size. I'd always used the excuse that I was far too big to be jumping around, but *Strictly* proved me very, very wrong.

Despite training for the show, it still took me a while to put on a pair of leggings and make a start on incorporating regular exercise into my life. I had such an 'all or nothing' attitude towards it. There was also still a bit of fear that it wouldn't work for me. I was dancing for hours and hours on end on *Strictly* and not seeing much of a change. Would going to the gym for an hour three times a week really make a difference?

As I soon discovered, yes, it would.

I was so overweight that when I started exercising I was beginning to doubt whether my body was capable of ever looking toned in any way. I was scared things had gone too far and that my body was ruined for life. Now I've got muscles in my arms I never even knew existed, and that's because I persevered.

I won't lie – because I never do! – I did really go for it from the beginning. I was doing uphill walks at 6 a.m., which I know is extreme. I'm not saying you have to do the same, but perhaps you could drop the kids off at school and then go for a long walk. Or walk to work instead of taking the bus? Or why not go for a bike ride? If you don't own a bike, maybe you could borrow one from a friend. Or some places will hire them. It costs £2 to hire a street bike where I live in London, and I know there are similar schemes in other parts of the country. You'll get fit and discover new things at the same time.

Don't let yourself sit for too long. Get up and walk around. People who sit down all day end up feeling more tired and sluggish. So many of us sit on our backsides far too much, especially if our job involves being at a desk. And how often do you spend hours lying in front of the TV at night? Never sit for more than an hour at a time without getting up and walking around or stretching.

Stop telling yourself you're tired. Tired people get tired. You become what you think. Of course people get tired – we've all got busy lives – but you can find the energy to work out. You can. I've been there. Don't kid a kidder.

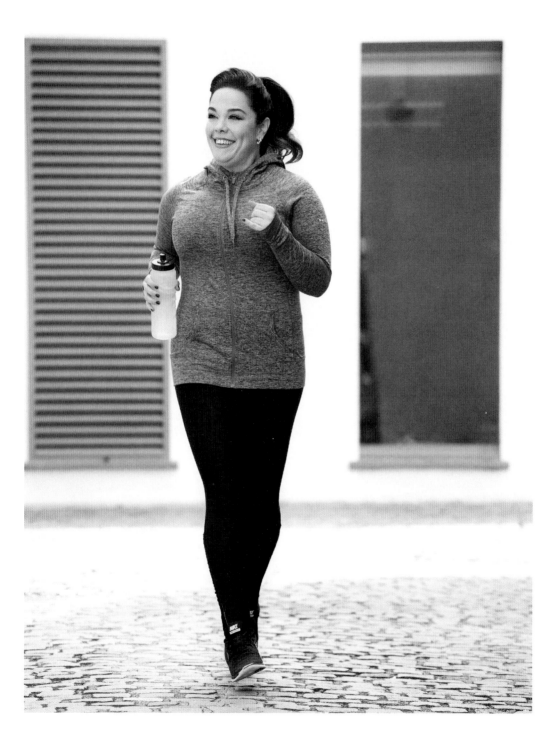

I know it's a cliché but walk up stairs instead of using a lift or escalator, stroll to a coffee shop that's a bit further away, borrow a friend's dog and do circles around the park. All these little things make such a difference.

You can do a half-hour workout in front of the TV every morning or evening while you're watching something, or walk up and down your stairs at home while you're listening to music. Small changes can get big results. Don't be put off by thinking you have to join a gym and pay hundreds of pounds for a personal trainer. You've got a mini gym in your own home. You just don't realize it yet.

YOU CAN DO IT!

I don't believe in 'can't, 'Can't' means 'won't'. I'm telling you:

YOU'VE GOT THIS!

I'm aware that impatience pangs could come into play again when you start working out, so I want to remind you not to expect overnight results. Please, please don't think you'll look like an Olympic athlete after two weeks of working out, because it doesn't happen like that.

But you will see changes, I promise, and the weight will soon start to fall off you.

As with healthy eating, please do not give up if you don't see immediate results. Changes are taking place – even if they're not visible. You've got so many small muscles that will be waking up and tightening, and one day you'll suddenly realize that your bum is higher, or your legs are more toned. It will just take a while for your body to catch up, because it won't know what's hit it!

Patience is so important when it comes to working out, but it pays off. If you give up before your body has a chance to adjust, you'll slip back into old ways and run the risk of becoming a statistic again. I'm saying this for your own good.

This plan may be the first time you've exercised for a while. But you can do this! I want you to aim for a minimum of forty-five minutes every day while you're doing the 8-Day Kick-Start, if you can. That section is definitely all or nothing. If you want to get to a great body, you've got to push through the pain (unless it's from a genuine injury, of course) and set yourself up for the rest of the plan. And the rest of your life, to be fair.

I'm not completely evil – you are allowed to rest in between exercises. It's essential you keep hydrated. But don't spend more time lying on the floor drinking water than you do working out! If you really feel like you can't keep going, you can have a small handful of grapes, raisins or frozen raspberries to help, but steer well clear of garbage-laden energy bars or drinks. And if you ever feel dizzy or faint, please stop immediately and seek medical advice. Exercise isn't meant to be easy but it certainly shouldn't damage your health. Make sure you are listening to your body.

I know that some of you may have active jobs where you're on your feet a lot, but I'm afraid that doesn't count towards your daily forty-five minutes. Your body will already be used to doing that level of exercise on a daily basis so you need to ramp it up and override what you're already doing. As I mentioned before, if you're new to exercise you can gradually work up to your forty-five minutes, doing it for a little bit longer each day. And if you want to break up your workouts into chunks, you can do fifteen minutes in the morning, fifteen minutes at lunchtime and fifteen minutes in the evening. But you still have to sweat each time!

YOU CAN ALWAYS FIND FIFTEEN MINUTES!

Whatever you do, don't hurt yourself. Push yourself, but listen to your body because it will tell you when things are starting to genuinely cause damage. Always warm up first and stretch yourself out.

I did a hardcore step class quite early on, and I really hurt my knees. I was in so much pain I couldn't exercise for a few days afterwards, which was really frustrating. I didn't make the same mistake again.

Please don't worry about how you look when you're working out, or worry that other people will think you don't know what you're doing. You don't need to spend a fortune on trendy gear. Wear whatever you are comfortable in. Everyone owns leggings and a T-shirt. Or you can even work out at home in your stretchy pyjamas. Who cares?

There will come a time when you'll want go out and buy some new gear to show off your fabulous new figure. I know you're probably saying to yourself, 'That's never going to happen.' But turn that thought around right now!

Your journey is no one else's business. Don't worry about the gymatrons with their perky ponytails, expensive gym gear and faces full of make-up. They're probably at the gym because they're bored. You're there to change your life.

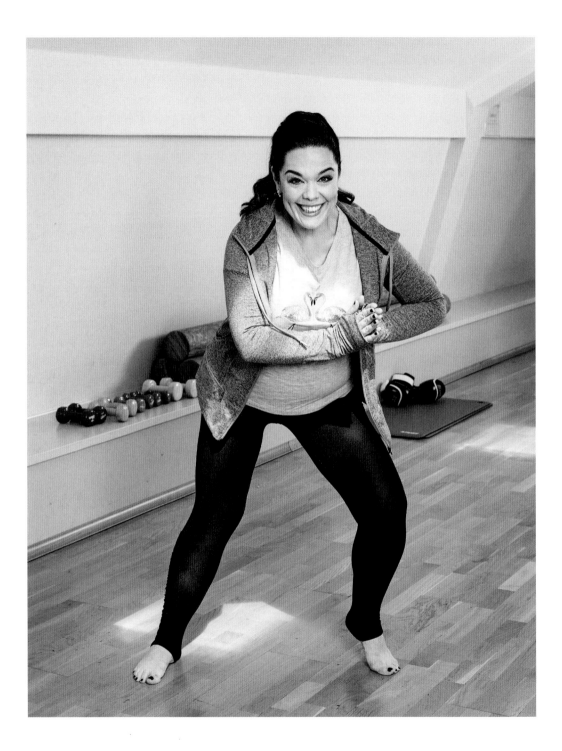

It's your yellow brick road, and you want to get to Oz. Let other people go on their own journey. Keep thinking about that moment when you're going to be able to fit into the skinny jeans in your favourite shop, or wear those old clothes you've been desperate to get back into. Think about that moment when you can phone a friend and declare, 'I'm in that bloody dress!'

If you like the idea of going to the gym and doing fitness classes, that doesn't mean you have to sign your life away. There are plenty of pay-as-you-go gyms around, or classes you can dip in and out of without agreeing to a lengthy contract. Lots of gyms offer free taster sessions. Or if a friend has membership, they can often bring a guest along for a day.

Also, if you really want to get some advice on your workout, pay around £5 for a day pass to a local council gym and ask a trainer for some advice. A chat costs nothing, and it's what they're there for.

You don't have to join a gym if it's not for you. Do a high-intensity interval training (HIIT) class at home in front of YouTube, or a really good DVD. (But choose wisely!) Set your phone and time yourself. No one needs to see you exercising if you don't want them to. Do it late at night or first thing in the morning, when everyone's in bed. Make this work for you. You could even start at home, and then go to the gym or local park as and when you feel ready, if you prefer to get your confidence up first.

Vibra boards, or power plates, are amazing if you're big. They vibrate while you're exercising on them and activate your muscle groups, which makes your workout much more effective in less time. Also, you don't have to move around much during the workout, which makes them really good for people who are very overweight. Most gyms have at least one, these days. If you want to invest in your own, you can buy them for around £100 now. I know it's more money to spend, so you could ask friends and family to give you a tenner each for your birthday and save up. Or put aside the money you would have been spending on snack food, booze or fags. You'll be amazed at how quickly you can afford one. And they work.

I used to swim all the time when I first started exercising and it's a great thing to do alongside HIIT and cardio. But swimming up and down at a leisurely pace isn't going to make much difference. You need to be doing front crawl, and you need to be doing it at a decent pace to get your heart rate up.

I also fell in love with aquafit and aquazumba. These are great for beginners because the water helps support your body as you learn to move around more energetically than you're used to.

Yoga is brilliant too. I know it's still got a bit of a hippy reputation, and you may not think it works your body especially hard, but it really does. Plus it's a great way to balance out your high-energy workouts. I'm not saying you can do it instead of cardio, but it can complement it. If I'm not working crazy hours I'll do evening yoga classes three times a week and it calms me down and rounds off my day. I sleep so well afterwards, too.

If you're too embarrassed to go to yoga because you're not sure if you'll be able to get into the positions, you don't need to go to a class with a fancy yoga mat. Put a towel down on the floor of your living room and watch a DVD or YouTube video. A lot of teachers also offer classes via Skype.

I completely identify with feeling uncomfortable and awkward in a class situation. When I first began yoga, even though I'm naturally quite flexible, I couldn't get into the poses because my massive gut got in the way. I was so ashamed. But things soon began to change.

Spin classes can be hard when you're big so I would start out either by riding your own bike, or by trying out the bikes in the gym to see if they suit you. If you find a class too painful there is no shame in leaving. I want you to be healthy and happy, not injured and miserable.

Personally, I *did* join a gym and I *did* go regularly. The very first thing I did was high cardio. It wasn't easy but I noticed a difference so quickly.

Don't get me wrong; I had my moments. Once, when I was getting ready for aquafit, I looked down at my thighs and they looked like a couple of monster chicken fillets (well, more like whole chickens) and I did not want to leave that changing room. But I told myself that I'd done it to my body and now I had to undo it. So I took a deep breath, walked out and did the class.

Did anyone turn to look? Maybe. Did it scar me for life? Absolutely not. And I felt bloody great once I'd finished.

I was very lucky that I could afford to get a personal trainer when I threw myself into exercise, but I found that a lot of trainers I met didn't actually know how to train obese or very overweight people. They're great with 'normal-sized' people or slim ones, but I was so far gone that no one knew what to do with me. That's when I had to do more of my own investigating to find out what I could and couldn't do, and what would melt my fat the quickest.

As is my way, I hopped online and researched for hours. The most important thing I learned, which is still serving me well, is that you need to sweat in order to burn fat. It's cardio all the way. Sorry!

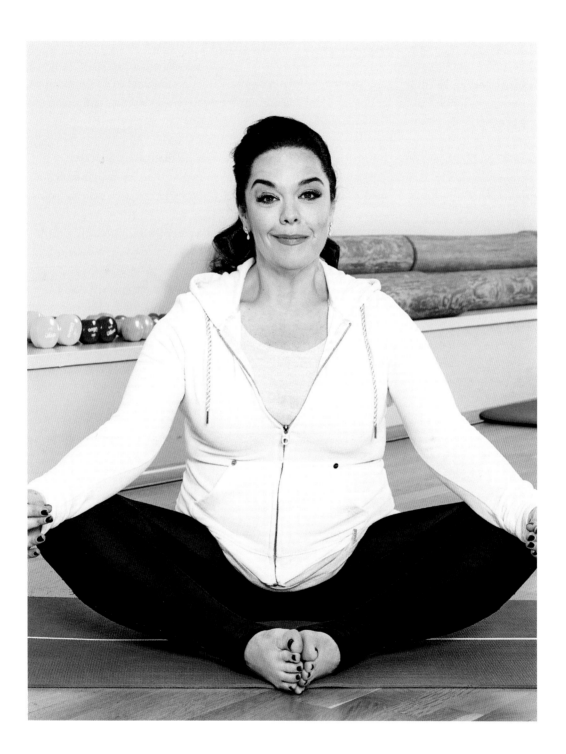

SWEAT IS FAT CRYING

If you're sweating you're going to burn fat. Forget 'glowing'; you need to look like you've done the ice bucket challenge. You're not going to look glamorous while you're working out, and you're not supposed to.

There is no point going on a treadmill and walking slowly. You can do that on a pavement. Get your heart going. Walk up hills and walk fast. I used to visualize 'slim Lisa' in my head and power walk towards her at breakneck speed (with the help of a good sports bra!).

Now, I must, must, must say this: Don't confuse cardio with running. People always think, 'I can't do cardio because I can't run.'

The good news is you don't have to run right now. Maybe later on down the line you'll do some HIIT-style running (where you run intensely for two-minute intervals), but no one is expecting you to start training for a marathon any time soon. I've been there, and there's no way I could have gone running with my fat jiggling around. It's only been in the last six months that running has become a part of my workout. Cardio is all about high energy. If you've got a lot of weight to lose, you're better off doing 65–70 star jumps than going for a run.

The two cardio classes I loved the most were boxercise and zumba. Both are great fun and make you feel unbelievable afterwards. If I ever went into a boxercise class feeling stressed, I'd come out feeling the opposite.

It's true what they say: exercise releases hormones that make you feel incredible!

If you're exercising in the evening, you must not go home and eat afterwards. This will make your workout pointless, because you'll be interrupting your body's fat-burning process. If you're training at night, eat something light a couple of hours before you go. Once you've worked out you need to be in a no-food zone, so load up on water instead.

Instagram, Pinterest, Twitter and YouTube are packed with advice and help. One of the things I loved doing right at the start was putting together a Pinterest page (it's free!) of inspirational photos and quotes to keep me going. Here's one of my favourites:

IF IT WAS EASY, EVERYONE WOULD DO IT!

As well as looking at other people's social media for inspo, the thing that's guaranteed to make me jump out of bed in the morning is looking at old photos of myself on my phone. I do it first thing every morning and, no matter how tired I am, it motivates me. I'm always one tap away from looking at the person I never want to become again.

I've also started taking photos of myself when I look and feel good. It feels great to scroll through them and smile; they're almost like a comfort-food substitute. You're not being vain by taking or looking at photos of yourself – it's for motivation. They really help to keep you going, and it's a great way of documenting your weight loss.

SOME MORE THINGS TO THINK ABOUT

- If you want to train with friends, go for it. Some people find it really motivational. It makes them more likely to get up and go because they're accountable to someone. And if you've arranged to work out with someone, it's harder to get out of it. Personally, I prefer to exercise alone – other than group fitness or yoga classes – because I don't think you work at your full pace while you're chatting. You don't want to be talking about last night's episode of *Corrie* when you've got a job to do. If you're next to each other on the treadmill, you're not going to push yourself as much.

- Playlists are key. Create playlists of all the up-tempo songs you love. Don't walk or saunter along to Ed Sheeran ballads. If you want to burn fat, listen to music that revs you up and makes you work harder. I've included one of my own favourite gym playlists on page 132 – give it a go!

- All personal trainers say different things when it comes to eating before and after training, but if I'm working out in the morning I prefer to have my porridge first thing, at least half an hour before I work out, so I've got that hit of energy. I need fuel to get me there, and it makes me work harder. I also think if you're so hungry you feel like you're going to pass out while you're exercising, the chances are you'll end up cutting your gym session short so you can grab food as quickly as you can. Use your common sense and don't overeat before workouts, though – it's not nice to have it sitting heavy on your stomach as you're moving around!

- Don't end your workout in the café. I see so many people who only go to the gym so they can eat a muffin afterwards, which will undo all your work and do more harm than good.

- Prepare to feel amazing after you exercise! When you exercise, your body releases endorphins, which boost your sense of well-being. Working out also suppresses adrenalin and cortisol, the hormones which cause stress and anxiety. So not only will training help you to look amazing – you'll feel fabulous too.

A NORMAL GYM DAY FOR ME

Bear in mind I've been exercising for some time now, and I've built up to this.

At the moment my cardio routine begins with ten minutes running on an incline on the treadmill, followed by ten minutes on the cross-trainer to warm up.

Next I'll do half an hour of free weights, which involves lifting dumbbells while doing squats and lunges. I have gradually increased the weight of my dumbbells, and I suggest you do the same, starting with the lowest and building up so that the weight is always manageable, but a bit of a challenge.

Most days I'll follow that up with:

- 3 x 1 minute of twist crunches with a 30-second rest in between each set
- 100 star jumps, followed by a 3-minute rest
- 3 x 1 minute in a plank position, with a 1-minute rest in between each plank

HOME IS WHERE THE HEART (RATE) IS

All you need for home workouts are a few props. This routine will definitely get your heart rate up and get your body burning fat.

You can mix and match these exercises, but do a minimum of forty-five minutes a day to begin with, eventually building up to an hour. Don't think you have to rush through everything. You only need to do that with the high-intensity exercises. It will actually be more beneficial to do things like squats and arm lifts in a slow and controlled manner, so you can experience the burn and feel them working. You're much less likely to injure yourself this way, too.

WARMING UP

- Grab a towel and stretch your body out on the floor (in preparation for the exercises to come).

- Stretch your arms and legs out as far as they can go, and slowly move your head from right to left and back again several times.

- Stand up and stretch your arms to the ceiling. Stretch each leg out to the side (one at a time, obviously – unless you have serious magic skills).

- Slowly bend over as far as you can, hold for 10 seconds, then return to a standing position.

- Stand with your legs a hip width apart and lean your upper body back ever so slightly, allowing your shoulders to drop. Hold for 5 seconds.

- Do 5 minutes of speed-walking on the spot, rotating your arms at the same time to get your heart going.

- You're good to go!

MY CARDIO PLAYLIST

These are the songs that motivate me to push myself even further when I'm working out.

'Need U' – *Duke Dumont*

'When a Woman' – *Gabrielle*

'Get On Your Feet' – *Gloria Estefan*

'Escapade' – *Janet Jackson*

'Marry the Night' – *Lady Gaga*

'Vogue' – *Madonna*

'All about Tonight' – *Pixie Lott*

'Born Naked' – *RuPaul*

'If You Really Loved Me' – *Stevie Wonder*

'Let's Groove' – *Earth, Wind and Fire*

'Finally' – *CeCe Peniston*

'Shine On' – *Degrees of Motion*

'Super Freak' – *Rick James*

'Tell It to My Heart' (remix) – *Taylor Dayne*

'Can't Stop the Feeling' – *Justin Timberlake*

'Look Right Through' – *Storm Queen*

'Mr Saxobeat' – *Alexandra Stan*

'Evacuate the Dancefloor' – *Cascada*

'Hush Hush' – *The Pussycat Dolls*

'4 Minutes' – *Madonna, featuring Justin Timberlake*

'Uptown Funk' – *Mark Ronson, featuring Bruno Mars*

'She Make Me Wanna' – *JLS, featuring Dev*

'Let's Get Loud' – *J-Lo*

'Bad Boys' – *Alexandra Burke, featuring Flo Rida*

'Sissy That Walk' – *RuPaul*

'Signs' – *Snoop Dogg, featuring Charlie Wilson and Justin Timberlake*

'Peace' – *Sabrina Johnston*

'Let Me Love You' – *Ne-Yo*

'Play Hard' – *David Guetta*

TIME TO GET PHYSICAL

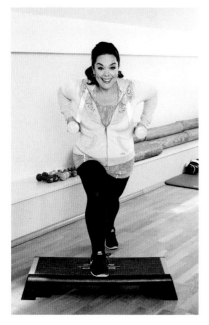

1. Hold one 2-litre bottle of water in each hand (or use light hand weights, which can be bought cheaply at Argos, Amazon or from some large supermarkets). Bend your arms and lift the bottles up 6–8 inches and then down again slowly until your muscles are complaining. Have a rest until your arms feel relaxed and then do one more rep.

2. Hold the bottles of water in each hand and do 20 squats. Do 2 more reps, resting for 2 minutes in between.

3. Keep hold of one of the water bottles and do 10 side stretches. Lift the hand holding the water bottle above your head and reach diagonally towards your opposite side so that you stretch all the way from your shoulder to your hip. Keep your other hand flat against your side and hold it there and slide it down as you stretch. Switch arms to do this 10 times on each side. Repeat twice, resting for 1 minute in between.

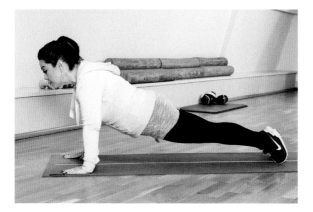

4. Hold a plank (where you are in a face-down position, resting on just hands and toes) for 10 seconds, then rest for 1 minute. Repeat twice more. You want to slowly build up your time (this is very important, because I don't want you to hurt yourself) so you can hold it for 1 minute, or longer. Then you know you're really fat burning. If you find the move too strong, you can drop to your elbows and/or knees instead of being up on your toes.

5. Speed-walk up and down the stairs for 3 minutes. Do 3 reps, resting for 1 minute in between. Make sure you're not wearing socks or slippery shoes for this one.

6. Do 2 reps of 20 opposite-knee-to-elbow exercises, a bit like a standing crunch, resting for 1 minute in between.

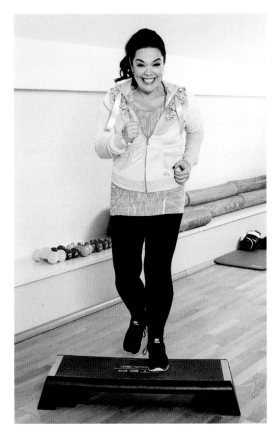

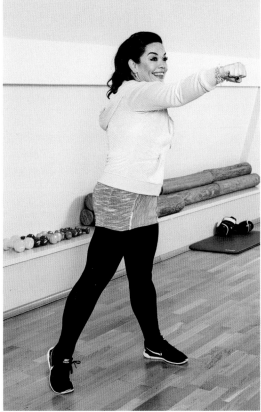

7. Climb on and off the bottom step of your stairs as quickly as you can, as if you were in a step aerobics class. Do 3 reps of 2 minutes, resting for 1 minute in between.

8. Punch the air in front of you as fast as you can for 1 minute. (Picture someone who's made you angry standing in front of you. It's a brilliant motivator.) Repeat 3 times, resting for 1 minute in between.

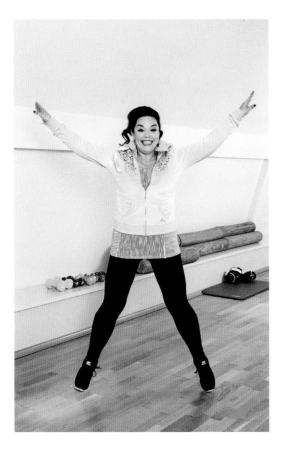

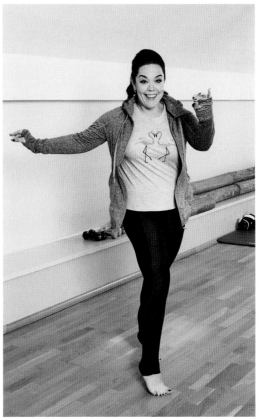

9. Do 50 star jumps at speed. Repeat 3 times, resting for 1 minute in between.

10. Full body twist with a lunge. Lunge forward with your right leg in front of you. At the same time turn your upper body to the right and move your hands as if you're turning a car steering wheel, so your left hand ends up in front of your face. Repeat on the other side. Do 25 on each side. Repeat again, resting for 1 minute in between.

11. Get zumba-ing. If you've done a few classes, you'll have picked up the basic moves. And they're so easy to do at home. Do 10-minute bursts of moves – such as jumping to the side and clapping, or some sexy salsa dancing. Then have a small rest before starting again! If you're struggling to remember sequences, look them up on YouTube.

12. Cool down by repeating the warm-up stretches, or doing some of the yoga moves on the next page.

YOGA

These yoga moves can be used as a stand-alone workout, but they're also great for helping your body cool down after training, and they're brilliant at preparing you for bed. I swear you'll sleep like a baby if you do some of these moves before you climb under your duvet.

Ideally, you'll build up to holding each pose for one or two minutes. Don't worry if you find doing just 20 seconds hard to begin with; it may just take a bit of time for your body to adapt.

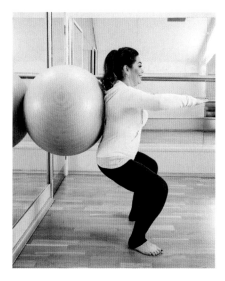

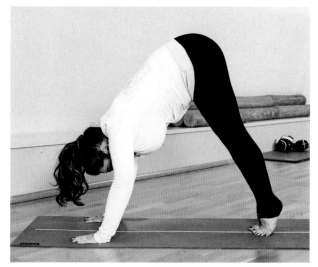

Get your kid's football or a beach ball from the pound shop. Or buy a cheap Swiss ball from a sports shop or supermarket. Put it between the base of your spine and a wall. Pop a good show on TV and slide up and down the wall, pressing against the ball and bending your knees into a squat, for 20 minutes. You won't even notice you're doing it.

Downward Dog. Go down on to all fours with your hands shoulder-width apart. Spread your fingers out widely so they provide a stable base. Curl your toes under and lift your bottom up in the air and slowly stretch your legs. Don't overstretch, though. Only push yourself as far as your body wants to go, and always keep a little bend in the legs. Hold and breathe deeply.

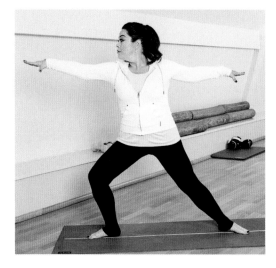

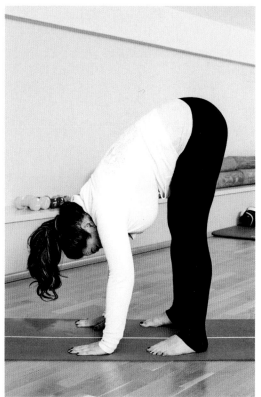

Warrior Pose. Step your feet wide apart, around 4 to 5 feet, ensuring your heels are in line with each other. Turn your front foot so your toes are pointing forward. The toes of your back foot should be pointing to the side. Roll your back foot slightly inwards to provide balance. Raise your arms to shoulder height and, with your palms facing down, bend your front knee so it is in line with the ankle of your front foot.

Sink your hips down as much as is comfortable, pressing down on the outer edge of your back foot to keep yourself stable. Keep your torso straight, look directly ahead. Hold and breathe deeply.

Touch your toes (I'm sure this move has a posh yoga name, but it does what it says on the tin). Stand up straight with your feet hip-width apart. Take a deep breath and lift your arms to the ceiling. Exhale and bend over very, very slowly, only going as far as your body wants to. Hold and breathe deeply.

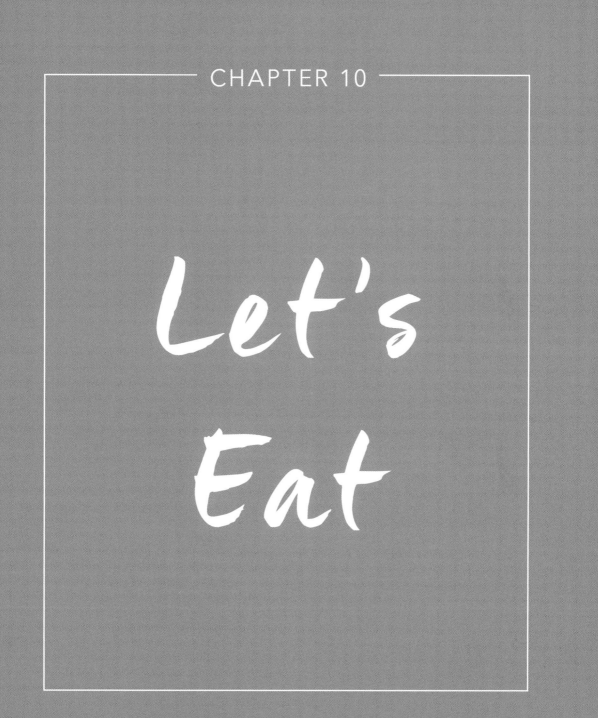

CHAPTER 10

Let's Eat

None of us have endless hours to spend in the kitchen (especially if you've also got a family to cook for) so I've kept my recipes as simple as possible. Some can be made in a matter of minutes, perfect for when you're getting 'hanger' pangs (hunger pangs that make you angry!). Some can also be adapted into larger meals for friends and family.

Make sure to record all your successes in your Honesty Diary, noting down which recipes work best for you and how you felt after eating them. Cooking is a great way of spoiling yourself and can be very therapeutic, so I really hope you love making and eating these dishes!

BEFORE YOU START

- My recipes and portion sizes work as part of this plan because they contain naturally healthy ingredients, and will satisfy while helping to shrink your stomach. Always be mindful, though. You must not overeat, no matter how healthy the food is, or you simply will not lose weight.

- I've included lots of soups and stews, because they're such a great way to nourish your body. They're filling, packed with nutrients, will help get your system moving and are easy to make in advance and take out in a Thermos flask, or reheat from the fridge when you need lunch fast.

- You'll even find some healthy takes on classic recipes that we all love, so you won't feel like you're missing out. There are pizzas and even chips on the following pages. But probably not like you've experienced before! These will be your saviours when you're having a wobble and feel at risk of grabbing junk food. Before you rush to order a Domino's or buy a ready meal, jot down how you're feeling in your Honesty Diary and make yourself work through those feelings. If it's comfort or nourishment you're after, plenty of the recipes in this book can provide that.

- All of the ingredients I've included are foods that you'll either have in your cupboard at home, or you'll be able to get your hands on easily. Don't worry! I'm not expecting you to go traipsing around looking for quails' eggs or coconut flour!

- One of the nicest things about losing weight has been discovering new foods I didn't know I liked, like scallops and quinoa, which are now two of my favourite things to eat. I've included some of my new finds in the recipes, but I've made sure everything is widely available and reasonably priced. If you don't fancy them, stick to my other recipes. I won't mind!

- If you're vegetarian and want to replace chicken with Quorn in any of the recipes, please do.

- You can cook your veg however you like, but the healthiest way is steaming because it allows the vegetables to retain the most nutrients. The steam bags you can get in supermarkets and most pound shops work a treat in the microwave, and take no time at all. Or you can pop your veg in a colander or sieve set over a saucepan of simmering water (cover with a pan lid if you want it to cook faster) until it's steamed to your liking.

- It's also totally up to you whether you want to use a regular blender, a stick blender or a high-speed blender like a NutriBullet to whizz up your ingredients where necessary, such as when making soups. They all do the job. If you don't have one already, most supermarkets sell basic stick blenders very affordably as part of their kitchen ranges, or you can easily get one online.

- It's always best to use fresh stock, if possible. You can get it easily in most supermarkets, but if it's not available – or if it's easier for you – of course it's fine to use cubes or powder instead.

- Where I suggest using lime or lemon juice, to make life easier you can of course buy it in a bottle. Personally I prefer fresh, but it's up to you.

- Another top time-saving tip is to buy jars of pre-prepared 'lazy' garlic, ginger and chilli. You can pick these up at many shops, and they save time and mess in the kitchen. But if you love chopping up fresh garlic cloves, go for your life!

STOCKING UP

Some things I always have in my cupboard to help me whip up quick meals and add flavour are:

Soy sauce	Lentils	Raisins	Mixed nuts
Dried chillies	Chickpeas	Oatcakes	Avocados
Garlic granules	Eggs	Bananas	Quinoa (either dried or ready-made in packets)
Salt and pepper (of course!)	Porridge oats	Coconut flakes	
Herbs and spices	Honey	Sundried tomatoes in a jar	
	Balsamic vinegar		

IMPORTANT!

You'll notice I have included potatoes in a couple of recipes, but these are strictly to be enjoyed later on, after you've reached your goal, once you're maintaining your new lower weight.

Ditto the coffee and walnut cake. That's your end-of-diet treat, and you're allowed to have a small slice. Just a small one! We've come this far, and we're never going back to our old ways!

As for the other desserts, they're not for every day, sadly. You can enjoy one of the sweet recipes once a week – maybe on a Sunday with the family – and always at the end of a meal, never as a snack in between. But certainly don't make them your staple.

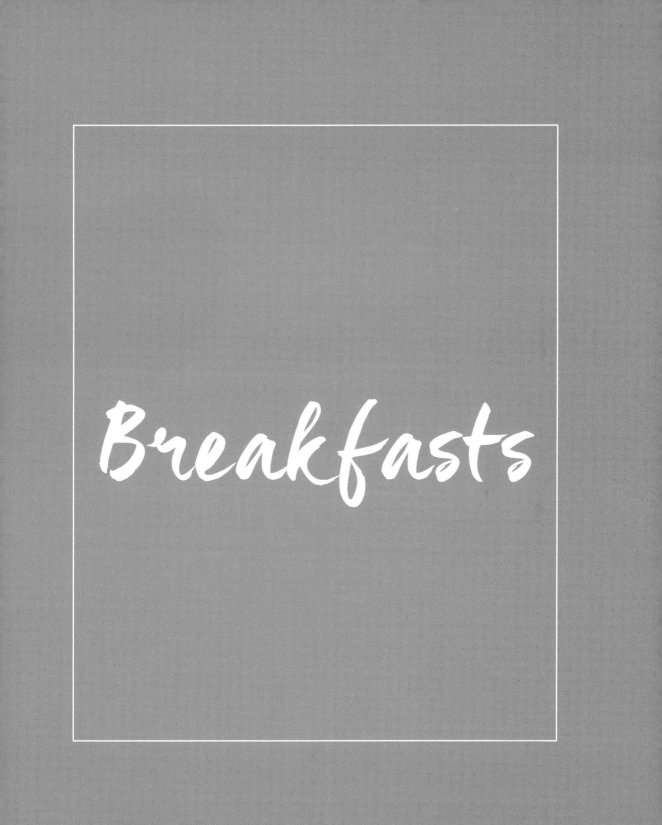

Breakfasts

STRICTLY HEALTHY PORRIDGE

This is without a doubt my favourite breakfast. When I was on Strictly Come Dancing, this is what fuelled my training! It made me realize how amazing porridge is, because even though I ate pretty badly during that time, I still had plenty of energy thanks to the porridge I had most days.

Serves 1

180ml semi-skimmed milk or almond, soya, coconut, oat milk

40g porridge oats

1 small banana or a handful of blueberries, or 1 teaspoon peanut butter

15g mixed seeds (I like to use linseed, pumpkin, sunflower and sesame)

15g raisins

1 teaspoon clear honey

½ teaspoon ground cinnamon (optional)

Mix the milk and oats in a pan and bring to the boil (keep an eye on it to make sure it doesn't burn or go sticky). Turn the heat down low and allow to simmer gently for 5 minutes.

Meanwhile, if you're having banana, chop it into small slices.

When the porridge is ready, stir in the banana, blueberries or peanut butter, along with the seeds and raisins. Transfer to a bowl and drizzle the honey over the top and finish with a sprinkling of cinnamon if you like.

Lisa's tip: Make up a big batch of your favourite mixture using 100g of each seed and keep it in an air-tight tub so that you can just take a scoop whenever you like.

Per serving (with banana) 478 cals | 17g protein | 13g fat (4g saturates) | 70g carbs (39g total sugars) | 6g fibre

CLASSIC GREEN JUICE

Before you flip the page, let me promise you that this is one of those recipes that may not look the prettiest but tastes amazing and does you serious good. People nag their kids to try new things, and now it's your turn. Trust me – you'll be glad you did.

Serves 2

1 apple, cored, peeled and roughly chopped

1 pear, cored, peeled and roughly chopped

Half a stick of celery, roughly sliced

Half a cucumber, peeled and roughly sliced

Juice of half a lime, freshly squeezed

4 ice cubes

200–400ml water, depending on how thick you like your breakfast juice

Pop all the ingredients in a blender and blend until smooth. And . . . you're done!

Per serving 63cals | 1g protein | 1g fat (0g saturates) | 12g carbs (12g total sugars) | 3g fibre

BURY BERRY SMOOTHIE

For this girl from Bury, it has to be berry! This smoothie is packed with goodness and gives you a real boost. You can drink it at home or on the go, and it's also easy to freeze so you can always have some in reserve.

Serves 2

250g frozen berries
250g low-fat yoghurt
50–100ml semi-skimmed
  milk
20g porridge oats
Clear honey for drizzling

Mix the berries, yoghurt and milk together in a blender until smooth. Add the porridge oats and mix well.

Pour into two glasses and drizzle a little honey on top for sweetness.

Lisa's tip: I also love making what I call a 'bung it all in' smoothie. This one isn't rocket science! Take any leftover fruit and seeds you have in your fridge or cupboard, add to some milk and yoghurt and blend until smooth. Literally anything goes. It's the perfect way of using up any leftover fruit that's nearing the end of its life.

Per serving (without honey) 171cals | 10g protein | 3g fat (2g saturates) | 24g carbs (17g total sugars) | 5g fibre

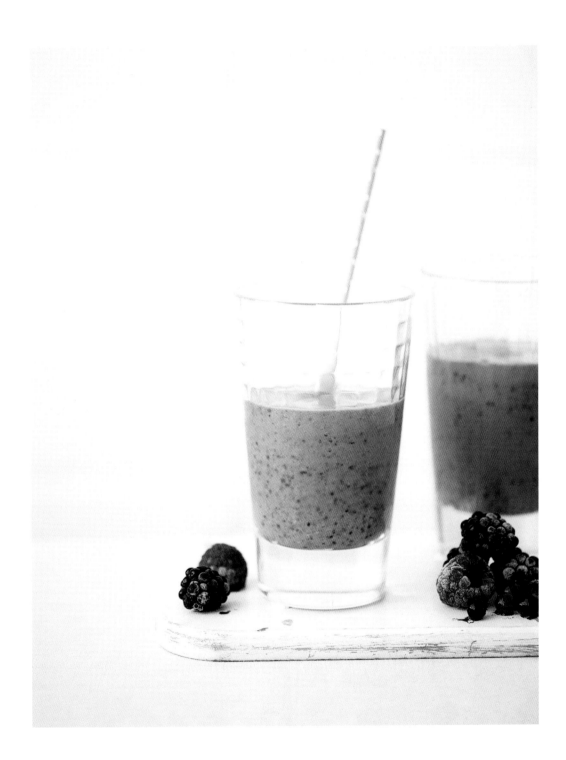

SCRAMBLED EGGS
WITH CHIVE, SPRING ONION AND AVOCADO

I eat this several times a week. It really fills me up and it contains a lot of protein, which is important for muscle strength when you're working out more often.

Serves 2

2 eggs

2 egg whites

2 tablespoons semi-skimmed milk

15g fresh chives

1 spring onion, finely chopped

1 teaspoon olive oil

1 avocado

Sea salt and freshly ground black pepper

Whisk together the eggs, egg whites, milk, a pinch of salt and a generous amount of black pepper. Stir in the chives and spring onion.

Heat the oil in a non-stick frying pan on the hob over a medium heat and then pour in the egg mix and reduce the heat. Stir continuously so it doesn't stick – the extra egg whites mean it wants to more than regular scrambled eggs. Cooking over a low heat makes the eggs lovely and creamy. Once they are cooked to your liking, remove from the heat and serve immediately with half an avocado, sliced lengthways, on each plate.

Per serving 204cals | 12g protein | 16g fat (4g saturates) | 2g carbs (1g total sugars) | 3g fibre

GRANOLA
WITH FRESH RASPBERRIES

Think about this delicious granola as your petrol for the day. Yes, I know you can buy granola in a box. But I really recommend making your own – you'll get so much more for your money, and you're in total control of what goes into it.

Serves 6

2 large egg whites

1 teaspoon almond
  or vanilla extract

3 tablespoons clear honey

2 teaspoons ground
  cinnamon

50g chopped hazelnuts

50g pumpkin seeds

200g oats

1 small punnet fresh
  raspberries

Preheat the oven to 160°C/Fan 140°C/Gas 3.

In a large glass bowl whisk the egg whites and almond or vanilla extract until the mixture begins to bubble, then stir in the honey, cinnamon, hazelnuts, pumpkin seeds and oats. Mix until all the ingredients are evenly coated.

Tip the mixture out on to a parchment-lined baking sheet and roughly spread out. Bake in the oven for 10 minutes. Remove from the oven and stir the granola mix to break up the clusters and make sure everything cooks evenly. Bake for an additional 10 minutes and then gently stir again. Bake for an additional 5 minutes or until the granola is golden and crunchy.

Leave the granola to cool on the baking sheet before adding the raspberries on top and serving.

Lisa's tip: If you have any granola left over, put it in an airtight Tupperware container as it should keep for a week or two.

Per serving 276cals | 9g protein | 12g fat (1g saturates) | 31g carbs (7g total sugars) | 5g fibre

SMASHED AVOCADO
WITH BABY TOMATOES AND HARD-BOILED EGGS

This is such a colourful breakfast. Who needs a full English when this quick brekky tastes so fresh and amazing?

Serves 4

4 avocados

200g cherry tomatoes, halved

4 hard-boiled eggs

Tabasco or chopped chillies (optional)

Sea salt and freshly ground black pepper

Mash the avocados on to four plates and season with salt and pepper.

Add equal amounts of cherry tomatoes to each plate and top with a sliced boiled egg.

Top with a dash of Tabasco sauce or some chopped chillies for an extra kick.

Lisa's tip: You can get cherry tomatoes in a whole array of colours, which is a great way to brighten up your plate.

Per serving 477cals | 11g protein | 44g fat (10g saturates) | 5g carbs (3g total sugars) | 10g fibre

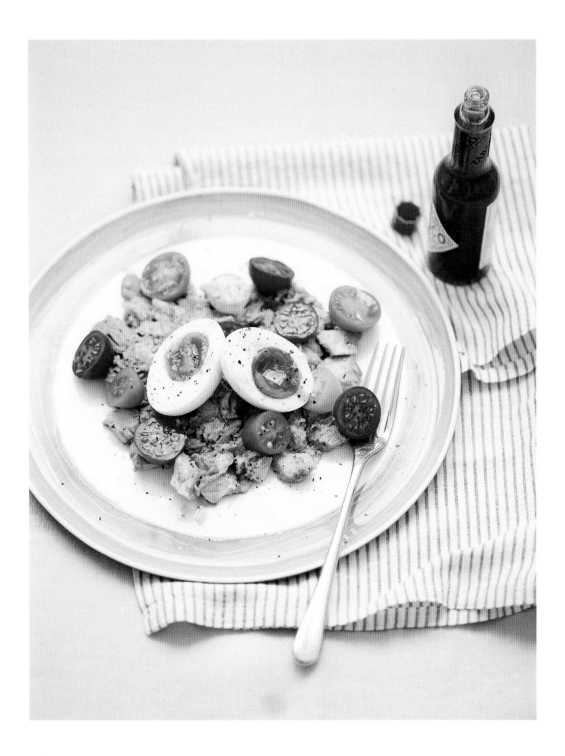

SMOKED SALMON
WITH ASPARAGUS AND BOILED EGGS

This is perfect for an indulgent Sunday breakfast in bed. It'll taste even better if you get your other half to make it for you.

Serves 2

12 asparagus spears
100g watercress
1 tablespoon olive oil
1 lemon, cut into quarters
150g smoked salmon
2 hard-boiled eggs, sliced
4 sprigs of fresh dill, stems removed, chopped
1 tablespoon capers
Sea salt and freshly ground black pepper

Boil some salted water in a saucepan. Add the asparagus spears and cook for 2–3 minutes. Remove and plunge them into cold water to prevent them cooking any further, then drain.

Place the watercress in a bowl and drizzle with the oil and the juice of two lemon wedges. Season with a little salt and pepper. Toss through to coat all the leaves.

Arrange the watercress on a serving dish. Lay the salmon over the salad leaves and top with the asparagus and sliced hard-boiled eggs. Sprinkle with chopped dill and capers, and serve with the remaining lemon wedges.

Per serving 288cals | 29g protein | 18g fat (4g saturates) | 3g carbs (2g total sugars) | 3g fibre

PIMPED-UP YOGHURT

Throw out all those artificially flavoured yoghurts and try the real deal. This is a hundred times better for you – and far more satisfying than any of the fruity yoghurts you can buy.

Serves 2

200g low-fat Greek yoghurt

1 fresh ripe mango, peeled and cubed

40g mixed nuts, roughly chopped (I like to use walnuts, cashews, pecans, hazelnuts and almonds)

1 tablespoon clear honey

1 lime, zest and juice

Fresh mint leaves, to serve

Divide the yoghurt and mango into two bowls. Sprinkle the chopped nuts over the top and drizzle with the honey.

Zest the lime over the two bowls, then cut the lime in half and squeeze the juice over each bowl. Decorate with a few mint leaves and enjoy the mouth-watering clash of flavours.

Lisa's tip: Make up a big batch of your favourite nuts, so that you can just grab a scoop whenever you need it.

Per serving 302cals | 14g protein | 16g fat (3g saturates) | 23g carbs (23g total sugars) | 4g fibre

CINNAMON BANANA POPS

These banana pops are fun, delicious and surprisingly filling. They're great for breakfast or as a healthy pudding. Kids will love them, too.

Serves 6

6 small bananas, slightly under-ripe
200g runny honey
Ground cinnamon and low-fat yoghurt or crème fraîche (optional), to serve

Peel the bananas and keep to one side.

Place the honey into a frying pan on the hob over a medium heat. Let the honey bubble and thicken and slightly darken in colour. This will take 4–5 minutes. Once it has reduced by about half its volume, add the bananas to the pan and carefully roll and turn them in the honey to fully coat them.

To serve, place each banana on a skewer and lightly dust with cinnamon if you like. You can also dip them into a little low-fat yoghurt or crème fraîche.

Per serving 183cals | 1g protein | 0g fat (0g saturates) | 44g carbs (42g total sugars) | 1g fibre

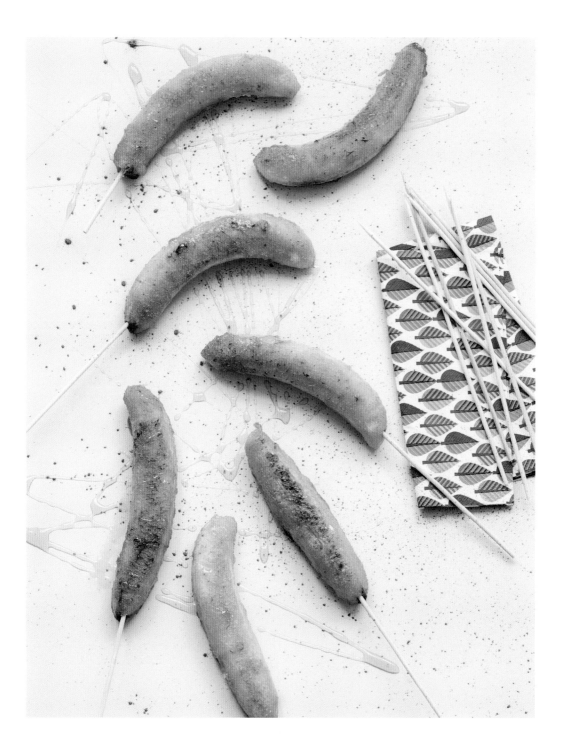

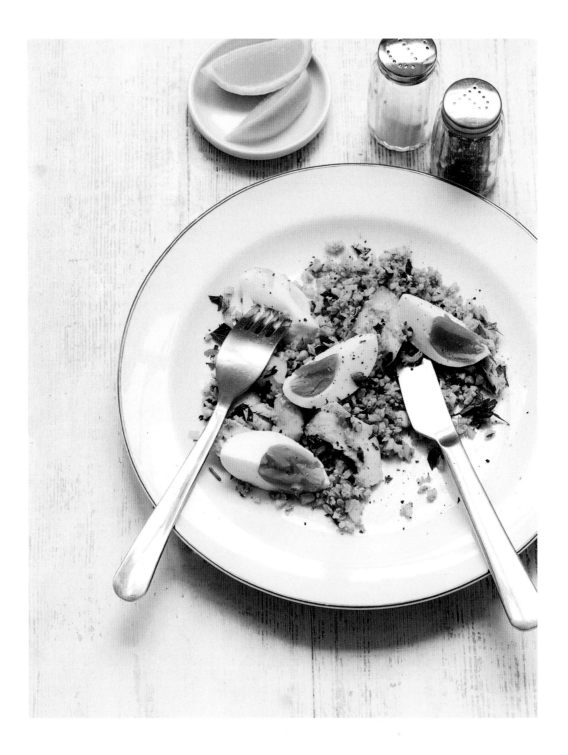

SUPER SIMPLE KEDGEREE

It's easy to get stuck in a breakfast rut, so here's a healthy, filling, wholesome idea you might not have tried before. Cauliflower rice is a simple alternative to rice — bigger supermarkets sell it in pouches. The smoked haddock adds a flavour hit that will tickle your palate and set you up for the day.

Serves 2

2 x 120g boneless, skinless dyed smoked haddock fillets

1 tablespoon olive oil

1 x 200g packet microwaveable cauliflower rice, or half a head of fresh cauliflower

2 tablespoons curry powder

4 tablespoons fresh flat-leaf parsley, chopped

2 hard-boiled eggs, cut into quarters

Sea salt and freshly ground black pepper

Brush the fish fillets with a little of the coconut oil and season them well.

Place under the grill and cook for around 4 minutes before flipping the fish over and cooking for another 4 minutes. Once they are cooked, set them aside to cool for a few minutes.

Meanwhile, microwave the cauliflower rice according to packet instructions. If you're making your own, grate the cauliflower using a grater with medium-sized holes so it's got a chunky texture. Then pop it into a microwaveable bowl, cover with cling film and cook for 3 minutes.

Mix the curry powder and the rest of the coconut oil together in a mixing bowl and add the rice and the chopped parsley. Stir well to make sure everything is evenly coated. Once the fish have cooled enough to handle, carefully flake them into the bowl and gently fold them into the rice and season to taste. Top with the egg quarters and serve.

Per serving 254cals | 33g protein | 11g fat (2g saturates) | 4g carbs (3g total sugars) | 3g fibre

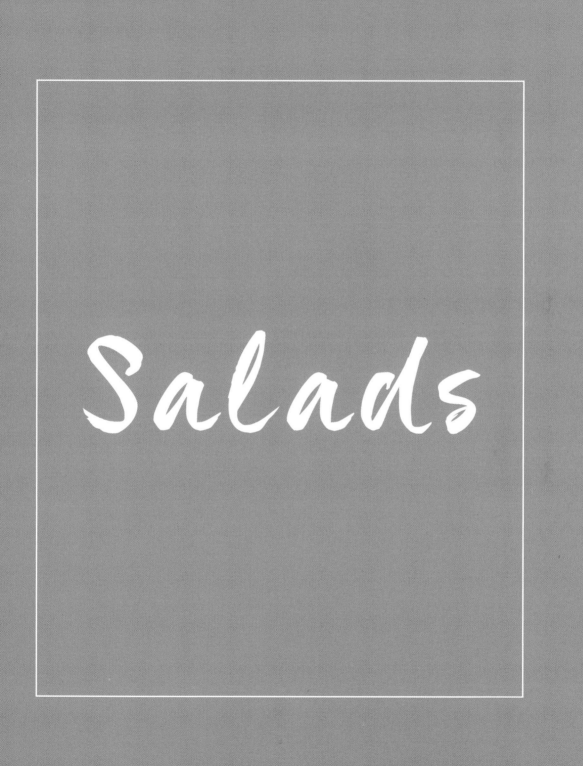

Salads

MY SUPER STRAIGHTFORWARD SALAD DRESSING

Diets generally teach us that salad dressing is bad, but it's especially bad when it's creamy and has a ton of added sugar. This healthier option is delicious – and you only need a splash to liven up a salad. It makes quite a generous amount, so if it's just for yourself then you might want to halve the ingredients.

Dresses 3–4 salads

Juice of 1 lemon
Juice of 1 lime
A drizzle of olive oil
3 tablespoons balsamic vinegar
Pinch of fresh coriander, chopped

Pop all the ingredients in a bowl and whisk. I said it was straightforward!

Lisa's tip: This will keep happily in the fridge for a day or two. I like to store it in a jar, so that it's easy to shake back up the next time I want to use it.

Per serving (per 1 tbsp) 18cals | 0g protein | 1g fat (0g saturates) | 3g carbs (3g total sugars) | 0g fibre

CHICKPEA AND AVOCADO SALAD

Chickpeas didn't use to exist in my world because I just had no clue what to do with them, but something changed and now I'm obsessed. They're dead easy to use – and so tasty. If you haven't discovered them yet, the time is now!

Serves 4

1 tablespoon olive oil

400g tin chickpeas, drained

1 tablespoon sweet smoked paprika

10 cherry tomatoes, halved

1 cucumber, sliced into half-moons

1 red onion, sliced thinly

1 large avocado, cut into chunks

2 large carrots, cut into thin strips

For the dressing:

2 tablespoons olive oil

Juice of 1 lime, freshly squeezed

½ teaspoon ground cumin

½ teaspoon chilli powder

½ teaspoon sea salt

½ teaspoon freshly ground black pepper

10g fresh coriander, chopped

Heat the oil in a frying pan on the hob over a medium-high heat. Add the chickpeas and the paprika. Toss to mix well and coat the chickpeas. Cook for about 5 minutes until the chickpeas turn golden brown and become a little crisp. Set to one side to cool slightly.

In a large bowl, mix the tomatoes, cucumber, onion, avocado and carrots. Add the chickpeas.

Place all the dressing ingredients into a bowl, reserving half the coriander, and whisk well.

Pour the dressing over the salad and stir well. Sprinkle the leftover coriander evenly over the top to serve.

Per serving 309cals | 7g protein | 21g fat (4g saturates) | 19g carbs (8g total sugars) | 10g fibre

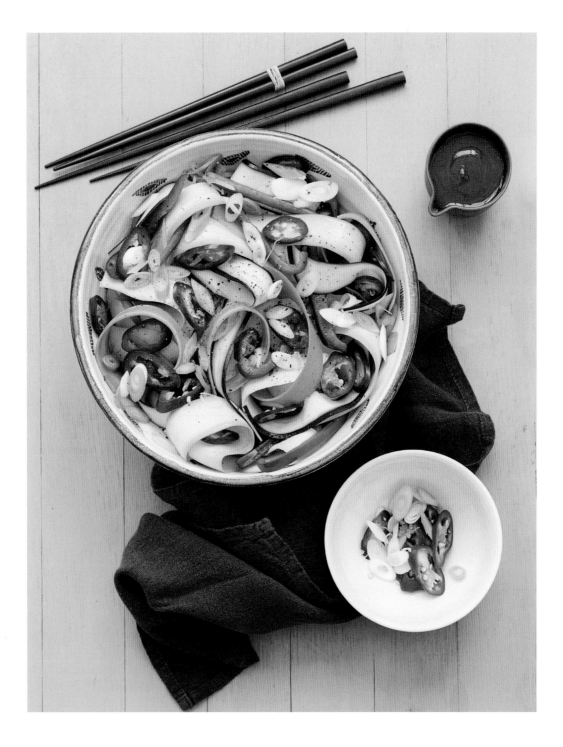

THAI COURGETTE AND CARROT SALAD

Not only does this zingy dish taste amazing, it looks amazing, too. Do I eat with chopsticks at home? Nope, you're far more likely to find them stuck in my hair and a fork in my hand instead. They look good in the photo, though!

Serves 2

2 carrots

2 courgettes (green or yellow, or a mix of both)

1 red pepper, thinly sliced

Half a red chilli, thinly sliced

2 spring onions, sliced on the diagonal

Sea salt and freshly ground black pepper

For the dressing:

2 tablespoons smooth peanut butter

1 teaspoon lazy garlic

2 tablespoons soy sauce

1 tablespoon clear honey

1 teaspoon sesame oil

1 tablespoon coconut oil or olive oil

Mix all the dressing ingredients in a non-metallic bowl or jug. Pop into the microwave and heat on full power for 30 seconds. Remove, stir and heat for a further 30 seconds. Set aside to cool down.

Using a vegetable peeler, create ribbons of carrot and courgette and place into a large bowl. Add the red pepper, chilli and onions. Season with salt and pepper and toss well. Add half of the dressing and toss to coat everything.

Serve the salad in bowls with the remaining dressing on the side.

Per serving (including dressing) 332cals | 10g protein | 21g fat (8g saturates) | 22g carbs (20g total sugars) | 8g fibre

CHICKEN AND MANGO SALAD
WITH CHILLI DRESSING

You may think it seems odd to put mango in a salad, but I absolutely love the refreshing contrast of sweet and savoury in this dish.

Serves 4

300g cooked chicken,
   sliced
2 mangos, peeled and
   cut into 1cm cubes
160g mixed salad greens

For the dressing:

2 tablespoons olive oil
3 tablespoons lemon juice,
   freshly squeezed
2 tablespoons fresh flat-leaf
   parsley, finely chopped
1 long red chilli, deseeded
   and chopped
Sea salt and freshly
   ground black pepper

Pop the chicken, mango and salad greens into a large bowl.

To make the dressing, whisk together the oil, lemon juice, parsley and chilli in a small bowl. Season to taste.

Drizzle the chilli dressing over the salad ingredients, and toss lightly to combine.

Per serving 231cals | 24g protein | 8g fat (2g saturates) | 14g carbs (14g total sugars) | 4g fibre

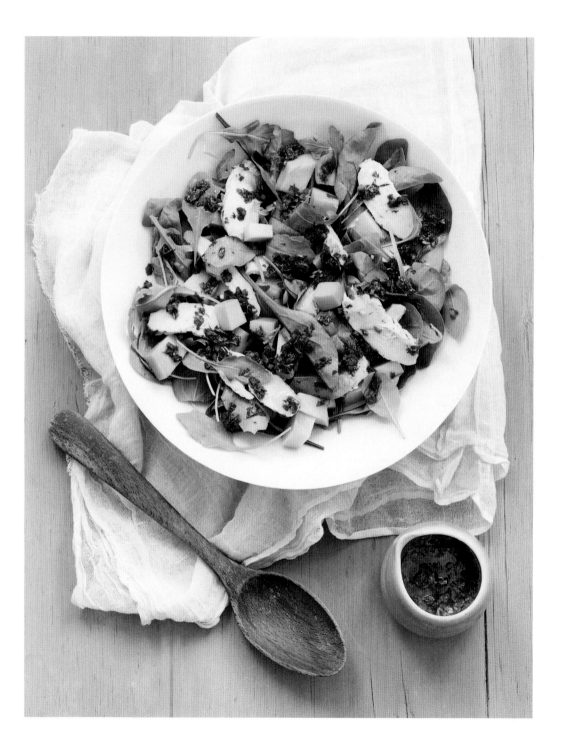

TOMATO, CAPER AND ONION SALAD

This salad looks so bright and colourful, and even though it has minimal ingredients it really packs a punch. Capers are like little flavour bombs that explode in your mouth. When recipes are this easy there is literally no excuse for not eating healthily!

Serves 2

5 large beef tomatoes, cut into quarters

1 red onion, thinly sliced

1 red chilli, thinly sliced

10 fresh basil leaves, roughly torn

Freshly ground black pepper

Mix all the ingredients in a large bowl.

Drizzle with my super straightforward salad dressing (page 160) and give the bowl a good shake.

Lisa's tip: Be sure to keep your tomatoes chunky to make the dish as satisfying as possible.

Per serving (including dressing) 144cals | 2g protein | 2g fat (0g saturates) | 26g carbs (24g total sugars) | 6g fibre

TUNA AND BEAN SALAD

This works brilliantly as a starter or a main, and it can be made in no time using mainly store cupboard ingredients. I will never get bored with this salad!

Serves 2

50g asparagus tips or tenderstem broccoli

Half a red onion, finely sliced into half-moons

80g spinach

160g tin tuna in spring water

400g tin cannellini beans, drained and rinsed

For the dressing:

½ teaspoon lazy garlic

2 tablespoons olive oil

1 teaspoon Dijon mustard

½ tablespoon fresh flat-leaf parsley, chopped

1 tablespoon white wine vinegar

Sea salt and freshly ground black pepper

Boil some lightly salted water in a saucepan. Blanch the asparagus or broccoli by cooking for 2–3 minutes. Remove immediately and plunge them into cold water to prevent them cooking any further, before draining.

In a large bowl, mix all the salad ingredients together.

Whisk all the dressing ingredients together until well combined, and gently stir through the salad.

Per serving 320cals | 26g protein | 13g fat (2g saturates) | 20g carbs (3g total sugars) | 10g fibre

LENTIL, FETA AND TOMATO SALAD

You can enjoy this salad as a main meal, or it also works really nicely as a small side dish alongside the chicken kebabs (page 200) or garlic and chilli prawns (page 212).

Serves 4

250g puy lentils

1 red onion, thinly sliced

4 large tomatoes, diced

25g fresh flat-leaf parsley, chopped

100g feta, crumbled

1 tablespoon chilli flakes (optional)

Sea salt and freshly ground black pepper

For the dressing:

2 tablespoons lemon juice, freshly squeezed

2 tablespoons olive oil

1½ teaspoons lazy garlic

½ teaspoon ground cumin

Rinse the lentils under cold running water and then place in a large pan of water on the hob over a medium-high heat. Once the lentils begin to simmer, reduce the heat slightly and cook for 25 minutes, or until they are tender. Drain and rinse under cold water.

Add the onion, tomatoes, parsley and feta to the cooked lentils, and toss to combine.

To make the dressing, place all the ingredients in a bowl and whisk well.

Add the dressing to the salad along with some seasoning. Add chilli flakes, if you want some heat, and mix well.

Per serving 349cals | 20g protein | 12g fat (4g saturates) | 35g carbs (6g total sugars) | 10g fibre

SPINACH, SWEETCORN AND FETA SALAD

I will never fall out of love with sweetcorn, and it makes a great partner for spinach, which is such a fantastic superfood. A word of warning: this dish isn't a feta free-for-all. You need to carefully moderate the amount you use – and don't keep picking at it once you've eaten!

Serves 4

160g baby spinach

3 large tomatoes, cut into slim wedges

200g tin sweetcorn

1 onion, thinly sliced

1 avocado, cut into chunks

1 green pepper, diced into 2cm pieces

100g feta cheese, crumbled

Sea salt and freshly ground black pepper

For the dressing:

See salad dressing recipe on page 160

In a large bowl, mix together the spinach, tomatoes, sweetcorn, onion, avocado and green pepper. Pour the dressing over the top and mix again.

Crumble over the feta. Finish with a touch of salt and pepper.

Per serving 262cals | 8g protein | 17g fat (6g saturates) | 17g carbs (13g total sugars) | 6g fibre

CHICKEN SATAY SALAD

This is a crowd-pleaser, so it's a great dish to make when people come round. But I know from experience that it's very easy to keep picking at it — so be careful you don't overindulge!

Serves 4

4 chicken breasts, skin removed

3 tablespoons Thai peanut sauce

1 tablespoon olive oil

2 tablespoons lime juice, freshly squeezed

2 tablespoons water

Half an iceberg lettuce, shredded

1 cucumber, cut into sticks

1 large carrot, halved and thinly sliced

1 red pepper, thinly sliced

25g fresh coriander, roughly chopped

Sea salt and freshly ground black pepper

Extra coriander leaves, to serve

Slice the chicken breasts into 2cm cubes, place in a bowl and coat with 2 tablespoons of the Thai peanut sauce, the coconut oil and salt and pepper. Pop the chicken under the grill on a medium heat for around 12–15 minutes, turning occasionally.

In a large bowl, whisk the rest of the peanut sauce, plus the lime juice and water. Add in the lettuce, cucumber sticks, carrot, pepper and coriander. Season with salt and pepper and mix well.

Separate out into four bowls, top with the chicken and add more coriander to serve.

Per serving 243cals | 30g protein | 9g fat (2g saturates) | 9g carbs (8g total sugars) | 3g fibre

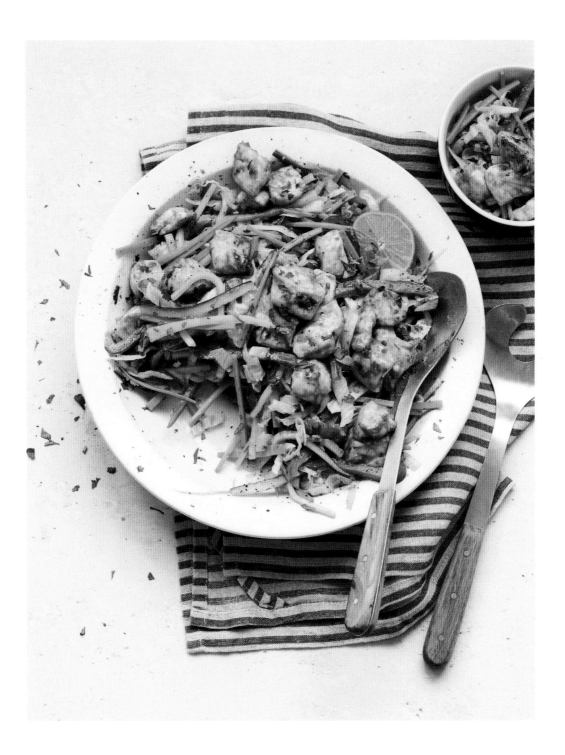

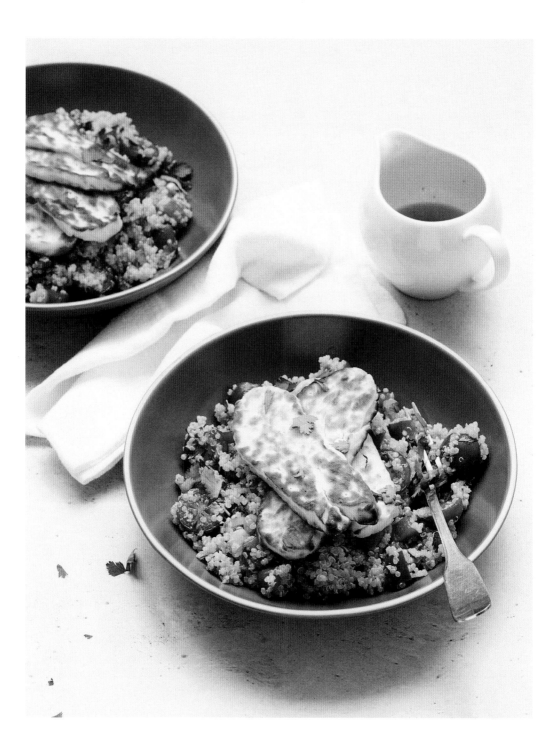

QUINOA AND HALLOUMI SALAD

Please don't be intimidated by quinoa — it may have a weird name, but it's honestly not as scary or posh as it sounds. It's super easy to cook, or you can even buy it in ready-to-use pouches. These days, you can pick it up anywhere. You'll be the queen of quinoa before you know it!

Serves 2

120g quinoa

6 slices of halloumi cheese

3 spring onions, thinly sliced into rounds

8 cherry tomatoes, halved

1 red pepper, diced into 1cm chunks

10g fresh coriander, chopped

Sea salt and freshly ground black pepper

Extra coriander leaves, to garnish

For the dressing:

1 tablespoon olive oil

Juice of 1 lemon, freshly squeezed

1 teaspoon clear honey

Start by cooking the quinoa according to the packet instructions. Once cooked, drain and transfer to a mixing bowl. Set aside.

Cook the halloumi slices under the grill for 4–5 minutes on each side, until the cheese is golden brown.

Make the dressing in a small bowl by whisking the oil, lemon juice and honey together. Season to taste.

Add the onions, tomatoes, red pepper and coriander to the quinoa. Add the dressing and combine well. Check the seasoning and add more if needed.

Divide the quinoa mix between two shallow bowls or plates. Place the halloumi slices on top of the quinoa and garnish with some extra coriander.

Per serving 527cals | 28g protein | 27g fat (14g saturates) | 41g carbs (12g total sugars) | 7g fibre

SESAME PRAWN SALAD

This is one of my favourite recipes. The soft juiciness of the prawns contrasts really nicely with the delicious crunch of the sesame seeds.

Serves 2

1 tablespoon sesame seeds

120g bag mixed salad leaves

10 tiger prawns, cooked and shelled

6 cherry tomatoes, each sliced into thirds

Quarter of a red chilli, thinly sliced

Half a red onion, thinly sliced

Half an avocado

Sea salt and freshly ground black pepper

For the dressing:

2 tablespoons sesame oil

Half a lemon, freshly squeezed juice only

1 tablespoon dark soy sauce

¼ teaspoon lazy garlic

¼ teaspoon lazy ginger

1 teaspoon clear honey

In a hot frying pan toast the sesame seeds until golden brown. Move them around constantly in the pan so both sides are cooked. Set aside.

Pop the salad leaves into a bowl along with the prawns, tomatoes, chilli and onion. Toss to combine and season well with salt and pepper.

Put all of the dressing ingredients into a jar, put the lid on and shake well.

Slice the avocado and add to the salad. Finish by drizzling the dressing and scattering the sesame seeds over the prawn salad.

Per serving 325cals | 13g protein | 26g fat (5g saturates) | 8g carbs (7g total sugars) | 5g fibre

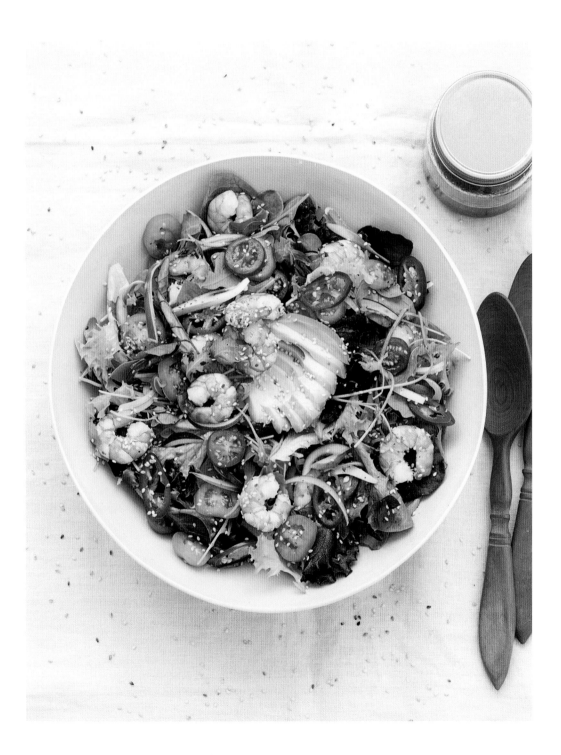

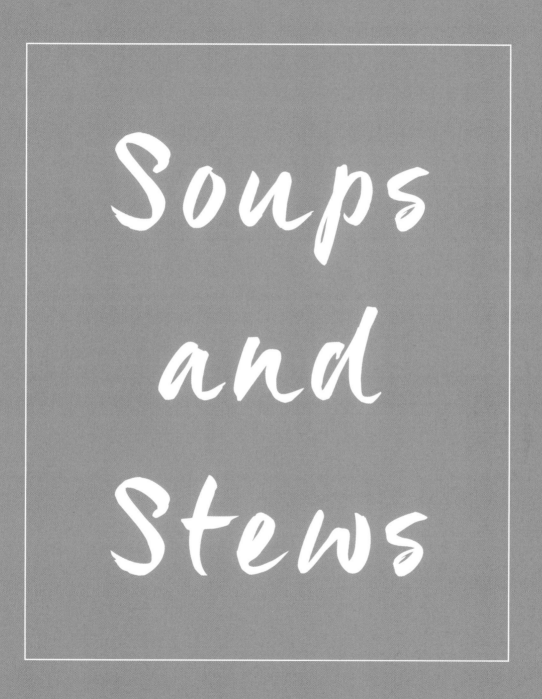

Soups and Stews

SIMPLE TOMATO SOUP

Ditch the Heinz, this soup is where it's at! It's a great one if you're ever feeling under the weather as it is packed with vitamin C, so it'll help you get back on your feet in no time.

Serves 6

2 tablespoons olive oil

1 large onion, chopped

1 carrot, chopped

1 stick of celery, chopped

2 cloves of garlic, peeled

800g fresh tomatoes, cut into quarters

400g tin chopped tomatoes

500ml fresh vegetable or chicken stock

20g fresh basil, chopped

Sea salt and freshly ground black pepper

A few fresh basil leaves, to garnish

Heat the oil in a large saucepan on the hob over a medium heat. Sauté the onion, carrot, celery and whole garlic cloves for 5 minutes. Add the fresh tomatoes and cook for a further 5 minutes until they start to break down and release their juices.

Add the tinned tomatoes and the stock and bring to the boil. Lower the heat and gently simmer for 20–25 minutes, or longer if you like a thicker soup.

Add the chopped basil and blend well. Season to taste, pour into six bowls and sprinkle with the fresh basil leaves.

Per serving 97cals | 2g protein | 4g fat (1g saturates) | 11g carbs (10g total sugars) | 3g fibre

CHUNKY CHICKEN AND VEGETABLE BROTH

Soups are such a great way of ticking the vegetable box and getting great stuff into your body, and this chunky broth is no exception.

Serves 4

1 tablespoon olive oil

1 large onion, roughly chopped

2 large chicken breasts, sliced into strips

1 green pepper, diced

2 small stalks of celery, thinly sliced

1 medium carrot, peeled and sliced into ½cm slices

100g medium open-cup mushrooms, sliced

500ml fresh chicken stock

1 teaspoon dried tarragon

1 tablespoon fresh flat-leaf parsley, roughly chopped

Sea salt and freshly ground black pepper

Heat the oil in a large saucepan on the hob over a medium heat. Add the onion to the pan and stir until it starts to become translucent. Add the chicken and stir until it is all opaque and sealed.

Add the green pepper, celery, carrots and mushrooms and stir-fry for 5 minutes.

Add the stock, tarragon, parsley and seasoning. Simmer with the lid off the pan for 15–20 minutes.

Per serving 157cals | 21g protein | 5g fat (1g saturates) | 6g carbs (5g total sugars) | 3g fibre

CHICKEN SOUP
WITH RICE VERMICELLI NOODLES

This delicious soup is light yet filling, with a lovely chilli kick.

Serves 4

550ml fresh chicken stock

350g chicken breast, cut into thin strips

1 teaspoon lazy ginger

½ teaspoon lazy garlic

8 shiitake mushrooms

50g frozen sweetcorn

2 tablespoons light soy sauce

2 spring onions, chopped

1 fresh red chilli, sliced

50g rice vermicelli noodles

In a large pan heat the chicken stock and add in the chicken, ginger and garlic. Simmer for 10 minutes.

Add the mushrooms, sweetcorn, soy sauce, and half the spring onions and chilli. Simmer for a further 5 minutes. Add the rice noodles according to packet instructions – usually they need around 5 minutes.

Check the chicken is cooked through, then pour into four bowls. Sprinkle the remainder of the spring onions and chilli on top to garnish.

Per serving 174cals | 25g protein | 3g fat (1g saturates) | 12g carbs (2g total sugars) | 1g fibre

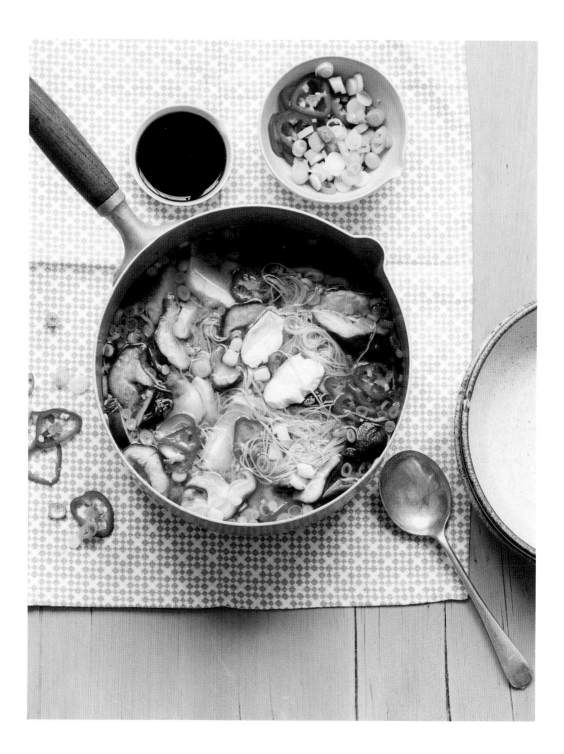

SAUSAGE AND BEAN BROTH

This is a really comforting, hearty meal, packed full of protein. Obviously it's a great winter warmer, but there's no reason why you can't eat it all year round.

Serves 2

2 sausages (pork/beef/
vegetarian, as preferred,
but make sure the meat
content is over 90%)

1 teaspoon olive oil

1 small white onion, finely
chopped

1 teaspoon lazy garlic

1 small celery stalk, finely
chopped

1 medium carrot, peeled
and finely chopped

400ml fresh chicken stock

Pinch of sea salt

½ teaspoon freshly ground
black pepper

1 sprig of fresh rosemary

210g tin butter beans

100g savoy cabbage,
shredded

Grill the sausages for 5–10 minutes until golden brown all over and cooked through. Set to the side to cool slightly.

Heat the oil in a large saucepan on the hob over a medium heat. Sauté the onion, garlic, celery and carrot for 5 minutes, then add the chicken stock, salt, black pepper and rosemary. Add the butter beans and stir well. Reduce the heat and simmer gently for 5 minutes. Add in the shredded cabbage and cook for another 5–10 minutes until the cabbage has softened and wilted.

Slice the sausages into half-centimetre pieces. Divide the broth between two bowls, remembering to take out the sprig of rosemary. Top with the sliced sausage, and enjoy!

Per serving (with pork sausages) 349cals | 18g protein | 18g fat (6g saturates) | 24g carbs (12g total sugars) | 12g fibre

BUTTERNUT SQUASH AND CORIANDER SOUP

I love, love, love this recipe. It's such a cosy soup, and if you ever feel like things are getting tough this will be like a massive hug in a bowl. I call it self-help food.

Serves 6

1 butternut squash
1 tablespoon olive oil
1 large onion, roughly chopped
2 sticks of celery, roughly sliced
1 teaspoon lazy garlic
10 mushrooms, cleaned and halved
1 litre fresh vegetable stock
25g fresh coriander, finely chopped
Sea salt and freshly ground black pepper

Preheat the oven to 200°C/Fan 180°C/Gas 6.

Top and tail the butternut squash; cut it in half lengthways and scoop out the seeds. Then slice each half into four wedges. Line a roasting tray with baking paper and place the squash on the tray. Roast with a sprinkling of sea salt for 40–45 minutes, or until you can push a skewer in with no resistance.

Heat the oil in a large saucepan on the hob over a medium heat. Sauté the onion, celery and garlic for 5 minutes. Scoop out the flesh of the squash from the skin and add to the pan along with the mushrooms and stock.

Bring the stock to the boil and then reduce the heat and simmer for 5 minutes. Season and blend until smooth. Stir through the chopped coriander and serve immediately.

Per serving 94cals | 3g protein | 3g fat (0g saturates) | 12g carbs (8g total sugars) | 4g fibre

SPICY CARROT AND LENTIL SOUP

As I've mentioned a few times by now, lentils are one of my favourite new discoveries. They fill you up so much – and they keep your body working as it should, if you get my drift…

Serves 2

1 teaspoon cumin seeds

1 teaspoon olive oil

2 carrots, finely chopped

1 celery stalk, finely chopped

1 small onion, finely chopped

1 teaspoon lazy garlic

½ teaspoon lazy red chillies

35g dried red split lentils

600ml fresh vegetable stock

50g low-fat Greek yoghurt (optional)

Handful of freshly chopped coriander leaves, to serve

Dry fry the cumin seeds in a saucepan, moving them around constantly so they don't burn. Add the coconut oil, vegetables, garlic, chillies and lentils, and fry for 3 minutes.

Pour in the stock and stir everything together. Bring to the boil and then simmer for 12–15 minutes, or until the lentils are swollen and soft. Blend until smooth.

Stir through the Greek yoghurt, if you want a creamier taste. Serve in bowls with the fresh coriander leaves sprinkled on top.

Per serving (including yogurt) 195cals | 9g protein | 4g fat (1g saturates) | 26g carbs 15(g total sugars) | 8g fibre

BUTTERNUT SQUASH AND RED LENTIL STEW

The word 'stew' often makes people think of meat, but this is proof that a veggie one can be just as delicious.

Serves 4

1 tablespoon olive oil

1 onion, chopped

1 teaspoon lazy garlic

1 tablespoon red Thai curry paste

400ml tin low-fat coconut milk

500ml fresh vegetable stock

1 small butternut squash, peeled and diced

350g dry red lentils

125g curly kale, chopped, thick stalks removed

1 tablespoon lime juice, freshly squeezed

Sea salt and freshly ground pepper

Heat the oil in a large saucepan on the hob over a medium heat and sauté the onion for 5 minutes. Add the garlic and cook for 1 minute more, stirring occasionally. Turn the heat up a little and stir in the curry paste. Mix everything together well for a minute or two – the paste should become very aromatic.

Add the coconut milk and stock, stirring well to bring everything together. Add the butternut squash cubes and bring to a boil. Reduce the heat, cover with a lid and simmer for around 15 minutes, or until the squash is starting to soften.

Add the lentils and continue to simmer for around 12 minutes until the lentils are al dente. Add in the kale and cook for another 3 minutes. Season and add the lime juice. Mix everything really well and serve immediately.

Per serving 504cals | 25g protein | 14g fat (7g saturates) | 64g carbs (13g total sugars) | 12g fibre

SWEET POTATO AND VEGETABLE CHILLI

I don't ever profess to be the best cook, but you cannot go wrong with this vegetarian take on chilli. Don't be afraid to play with flavour and add some extra vegetables or spices, if you want to.

Serves 4

2 tablespoons olive oil

1 onion, finely chopped

Half a celery stalk, finely chopped

1 teaspoon lazy red chilli

1 teaspoon lazy garlic

150g sweet potato, diced into 1cm pieces

1 tablespoon tomato purée

2 x 400g tins chopped tomatoes

70g frozen sweetcorn

½ teaspoon ground cinnamon

½ teaspoon ground coriander

½ teaspoon ground cumin

150ml fresh vegetable stock

Sea salt and freshly ground black pepper

40g low-fat Greek yoghurt and freshly chopped coriander leaves, to serve

Heat the oil in a saucepan on the hob over a medium heat. Sauté the onion, celery and chilli until they start to soften. After 5 minutes or so add the garlic followed by the sweet potato.

Add the tomato purée and stir well. Cook for 2 minutes before adding the tinned tomatoes, sweetcorn, spices and stock to the saucepan. Bring to the boil and then simmer on the lowest heat setting for an hour, stirring well every 15 minutes. Season to taste.

Serve topped with a spoonful of the yoghurt and a sprinkle of fresh coriander.

Per serving 170cals | 5g protein | 7g fat (1g saturates) | 21g carbs (13g total sugars) | 4g fibre

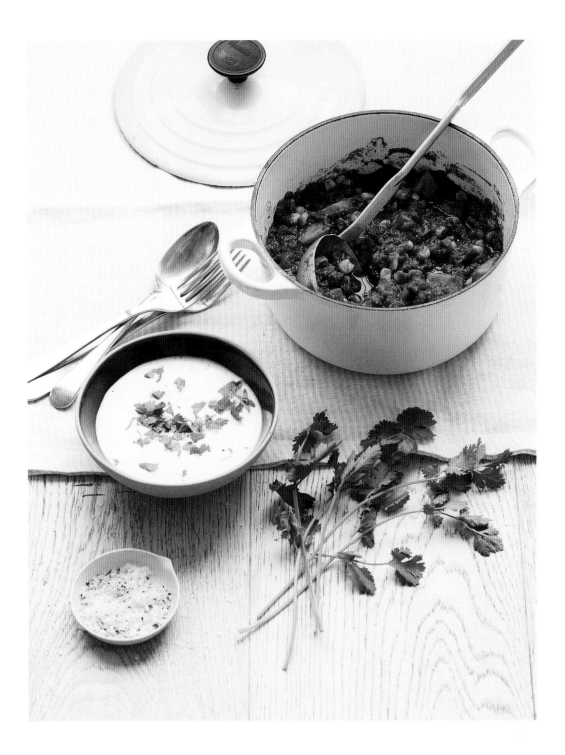

SPICY VEGETABLE CURRY

This is your very own – healthier! – version of an Indian takeaway. If the rest of your family are having a takeaway, you could even pop this in a foil container to give it an authentic look so you don't feel like you're missing out.

Serves 4

2 teaspoons olive oil

1 onion, chopped

500g sweet potatoes, diced into 1–2cm chunks

1 aubergine, diced into 2cm chunks

2 carrots, peeled and thinly sliced

1 teaspoon lazy garlic

2 tablespoons Rogan Josh curry paste

1 x 680ml jar tomato passata

2 courgettes, sliced into half-moons

200g green beans

Sea salt and freshly ground black pepper

25g freshly chopped coriander, to serve

Heat the coconut oil in a large saucepan on the hob over a medium heat. Sauté the onion, sweet potatoes and aubergine for 10–12 minutes until they start to soften and take on a little colour. Keep stirring as the starch in the potato will make it want to stick to the pan. Add the carrots, garlic and curry paste, and season well. Cook, stirring frequently, for 1–2 minutes, until the ingredients are completely mixed together.

Add the passata and then rinse the jar with a little water and add that to the pan too. Add the courgettes and green beans and continue to cook, stirring occasionally, for 15 minutes, or until slightly thickened.

Adjust the seasoning to taste, and serve sprinkled with the fresh coriander.

Per serving 274cals | 8g protein | 5g fat (2g saturates) | 43g carbs (22g total sugars) | 14g fibre

CHICKPEA AND LENTIL (SOPHIE) DHAL

Your mouth won't know what's hit it when you try this. It's unbelievable. I make it for friends, and they can't believe it's healthy because it's so wonderful and rich. Serious supermodel food!

Serves 4

250g puy lentils

1 tablespoon olive oil

1 medium onion, peeled and diced

1 red pepper, deseeded and diced

1 teaspoon lazy garlic

2 teaspoons ground ginger

2 teaspoons red Thai curry paste

400g tin chopped tomatoes

300g fresh spinach

1 x 400g tin chickpeas, drained

Sea salt and freshly ground black pepper

100g low-fat yoghurt, to serve

Rinse the lentils under cold running water and then place in a large pan of water on the hob over a medium-high heat. Once the lentils begin to simmer, reduce the heat slightly and cook for 25 minutes, or until they are tender. Drain and rinse under running water. Set aside.

Heat the oil in a large saucepan on the hob over a medium heat. Add the onion and red pepper and cook for around 5 minutes until the onion is translucent. Add the garlic and ginger and cook for 1 minute.

Next add the curry paste and cook for about 2 minutes, stirring all the time. Add the tomatoes, spinach, cooked lentils and chickpeas and stir to combine.

Continue to cook, stirring occasionally, for 10 minutes until the sauce thickens slightly. Season to taste. Remove from the heat, divide between four bowls and serve topped with a dollop of yoghurt.

Per serving 397cals | 25g protein | 7g fat (1g saturates) | 50g carbs (11g total sugars) | 16g fibre

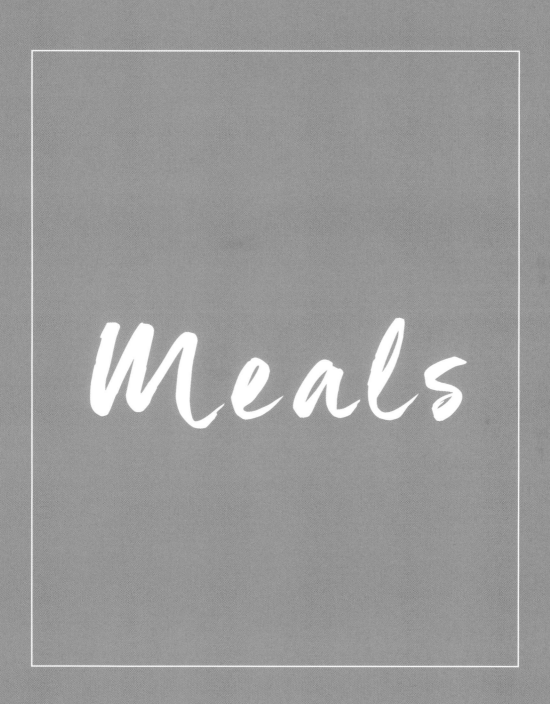

Meals

JALAPEÑO HUMMUS
WITH CRUNCHY VEG

If you want to stick to your diet, it's important to keep food exciting, and experimenting with spice is a great way to do it. This is the kind of food I'll box up and take with me when I'm on the road.

Serves 8

For the hummus:

400g tin chickpeas, drained

2 fresh jalapeño peppers, sliced (deseeded if you don't want it too hot)

3 tablespoons tahini

1 clove garlic, peeled and roughly chopped

Juice of 2 lemons, freshly squeezed

3 tablespoons water

Sea salt and freshly ground black pepper

For the veg:

4 large carrots, peeled and sliced into sticks

2 sticks of celery, sliced

10 cherry tomatoes, halved

1 red, 1 green and 1 yellow pepper, deseeded and cut into strips

1 cucumber, peeled and sliced into sticks

Whizz the chickpeas, jalapeños, tahini, garlic, lemon juice and water together in a food processor until smooth, which will take 2–3 minutes. Scrape down the sides and blitz for another minute. Add a little more water if it seems either too thick or dry. Season with salt and pepper.

Serve with the crunchy veg.

Per serving (hummus only) 77cals | 4g protein | 4g fat (1g saturates) | 5g carbs (0g total sugars) | 2g fibre
Per serving (including veg) 123cals | 5g protein | 5g fat (1g saturates) | 12g carbs (7g total sugars) | 6g fibre

STEAK AND VEGETABLE CANAPÉS

These rolled-up canapés look like something you'd get in a posh restaurant, but you can make them in minutes. They'll satisfy your hunger and impress all your friends. Win-win.

Serves 8

1 x 225g sirloin or flank steak (approximate weight)

2 tablespoons olive oil

1 sprig of fresh rosemary, leaves removed and chopped

1 red pepper, sliced into thin strips

1 green pepper, sliced into thin strips

1 medium courgette, thinly sliced

1 medium onion, halved and thinly sliced

3 portobello mushrooms, cut into thin strips

1 red chilli, cut in half lengthways, then thinly sliced into long lengths (optional)

Sea salt and freshly ground black pepper

Trim the steak of any fat. Rub each side of the steak with one tablespoon of the oil and sprinkle with salt, pepper and the rosemary.

Heat a frying pan on the hob over a medium-high heat, add the steak and cook for 3 minutes on each side. Remove from the pan and set aside on a chopping board to rest (cook for longer if you prefer your meat well done).

Heat the remaining tablespoon of oil in the same pan and cook the vegetables until tender. You want them to hold their shape and still be crisp – this should take around 4 minutes. Season with salt and pepper.

Carve the steak into half-centimetre slices and lay the slices out. Place a few of the vegetable strips (and the chilli, if you're using it) vertically on the end of each one. Roll the steak so the vegetables are sticking out of each end, and secure with a toothpick.

Per serving 84cals | 8g protein | 4g fat (1g saturates) | 3g carbs (3g total sugars) | 2g fibre

VEGETABLE FRITTATA

If you love quiche, which was a big part of my old diet, this is the perfect crust-free alternative. It's also one of those dishes you can bung any leftover veg into, so that nothing goes to waste.

Serves 4

1 red pepper
1 teaspoon olive oil
1 large onion, chopped
6 large eggs
300g low-fat natural
   cottage cheese
½ teaspoon lazy garlic
20g Parmesan cheese,
   finely grated
15g fresh flat-leaf
   parsley, chopped
100g leaf spinach,
   finely chopped
¼ teaspoon nutmeg
100g cherry tomatoes,
   sliced
4 asparagus spears,
   pre-boiled for 3 minutes
Pinch of salt
Freshly ground black
   pepper
Extra parsley (optional),
   to garnish

Preheat the oven to 230°C/Fan 210°C/Gas 7.

Roast the whole pepper in the oven for 20 minutes, turning once halfway through. Once the skin has started to blacken, place the pepper into a plastic food bag, knot the top and allow it to cool a little. Once you can handle the pepper, remove the pepper from the bag and peel off the skin. Tear the flesh into strips and keep to one side.

Heat the oil in a frying pan on the hob over a medium heat, and sauté the onion.

In a large bowl beat the eggs with the cottage cheese. Add the garlic, half the Parmesan, the sautéd onion, parsley, spinach, roasted pepper and nutmeg. Season with a pinch of salt and some black pepper. Tip into either a rectangular cake tin or an ovenproof frying pan. Top with the tomatoes and asparagus spears, and sprinkle the remaining Parmesan over the top.

Reduce the oven temperature to 190°C/Fan 170°C/Gas 5. Cook the frittata for 20–25 minutes until set. The edges should be slightly puffed and the top golden brown. Cut into wedges and serve hot, or cool down and store in the fridge. Sprinkle with additional parsley, if required.

Per serving 266cals | 22g protein | 15g fat (6g saturates) | 8g carbs (7g total sugars) | 3g fibre

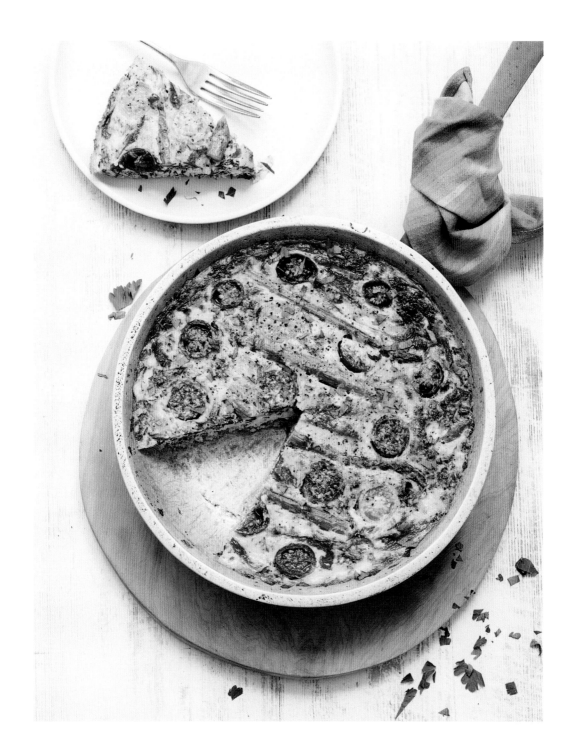

RED PEPPER AND MUSHROOM OMELETTE MUFFINS

I swear these are the healthiest muffins you'll ever come across, and you can add in any veg you fancy to ramp up the goodness. They're a great way to use up leftovers from your vegetable drawer.

Makes 12 muffins

1 tablespoon olive oil, plus extra for greasing

6 medium-sized mushrooms, diced

2 red peppers, deseeded and diced

1 large red onion, chopped

½ teaspoon garlic powder

8 large eggs

Sea salt and freshly ground black pepper

Preheat the oven to 160°C/Fan 140°C/Gas 3.

Heat the oil in a large frying pan on the hob over a medium heat. Sauté the mushrooms, peppers and onion for about 4–5 minutes until soft, then stir in the garlic powder and remove from the heat.

In a bowl whisk the eggs together and then add the mushrooms, peppers and onions. Season to taste. Stir well to coat everything in the egg mixture.

Grease a 12-hole muffin tin. Pour in the egg mixture, taking care to divide it equally between the holes and filling each one up about three-quarters of the way. Place the muffin tin in the oven and bake for approximately 20 minutes.

Remove and serve immediately, or let cool and refrigerate.

Per serving 73cals | 6g protein | 5g fat (1g saturates) | 2g carbs (2g total sugars) | 1g fibre

ONION OMELETTE

Don't worry about trying to make the perfect omelette. The onions here are so flavoursome, it will taste good whatever it looks like. This meal is also great for (ahem) helping to keep your bodily functions working as they should.

Serves 2

1 tablespoon olive oil, plus extra for frying

1 large onion, finely chopped

2 large tomatoes, diced

5 large eggs

¼ teaspoon sea salt

Freshly ground black pepper

Salad leaves, to serve

Heat the oil in a large pan on the hob over a medium heat. Add the onion and cook for 2 minutes or until soft, stirring frequently. Add the tomatoes and cook for another minute, stirring frequently. Remove half of the mix and keep to one side.

In a bowl whisk together the eggs, salt and pepper.

Add another teaspoon of oil to the pan. Pour in half the egg mixture and stir it around the pan to coat the onion and tomato, then even it out across the pan. Cook for around 2 minutes, until the edges of the omelette begin to set.

Once the middle of the omelette is just set, carefully fold it in half using a spatula and slide it on to a plate. Repeat for the remaining ingredients.

Season the omelettes with black pepper, and serve them with a green salad.

Per serving 293cals | 20g protein | 19g fat (5g saturates) | 9g carbs (7g total sugars) | 3g fibre

SKINNY TURKEY BURGERS
WITH CELERIAC CHIPS

Who says you can't have burger and chips on a diet? This is the kind of meal you can feed to your entire family and you won't hear a single word of complaint. Celeriac chips may not be the norm but they're such a winner.

Serves 4

For the burgers:

250g minced turkey

3 spring onions,
    finely chopped

1 teaspoon lazy garlic

2 sundried tomatoes,
    finely chopped

1 tablespoon fresh flat-leaf
    parsley, finely chopped

1 tablespoon fresh thyme,
    finely chopped

1 teaspoon olive oil,
    for grilling

Lettuce leaves and slices
    of tomato and onion,
    for topping

For the chips:

2 large celeriac

3 tablespoons olive oil

1 tablespoon mild
    curry powder

½ teaspoon sea salt

Preheat the oven to 230°C/Fan 210°C/ Gas 7.

Mix all the burger ingredients, except for the olive oil, together in a large bowl. Divide the mixture into four equal amounts and shape into burgers. Place them on a plate, cover and chill in the fridge for 30 minutes.

Peel the celeriac by slicing off the top and bottom and using a sharp knife to remove the tough skin. Cut into fat chips. Blanch the chips by boiling them, uncovered, for 2 minutes.

Drain the chips and then place them back in the saucepan. Add the oil, curry powder and sea salt, and coat the chips well.

Spread the chips on to a large baking tray, leaving space between them. Cook in the oven for 30–35 minutes until golden brown and cooked through.

Remove the burgers from the fridge and brush with the olive oil. Place under a preheated grill and cook for 3–4 minutes on each side. Dress your burger with the lettuce, tomato and onion.

Per serving 257cals | 21g protein | 14g fat (3g saturates) | 6g carbs (4g total sugars) | 11g fibre

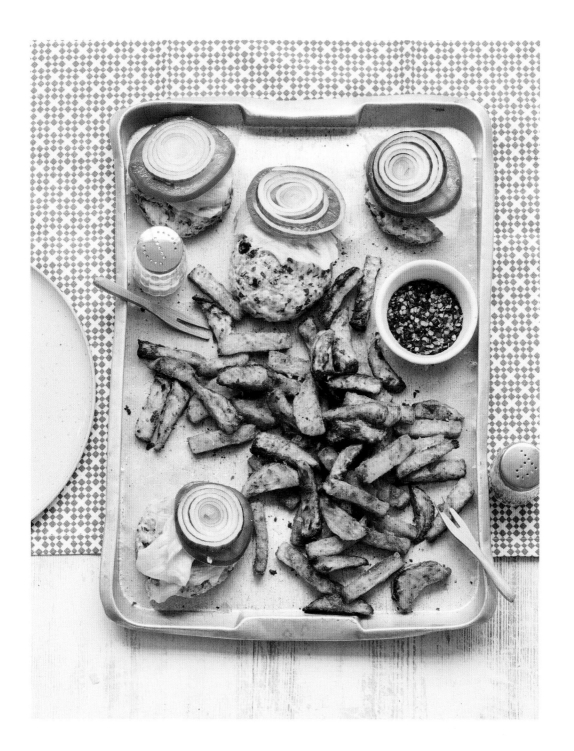

ROSEMARY, LEMON CHICKEN AND VEGETABLE KEBABS

The rosemary and lemon in this recipe provide such fragrant flavours. Rosemary is a herb I use a lot these days, and I've learned from experience that a little goes a really long way.

Serves 4

2 chicken breasts, cut into 4cm pieces

1 red pepper, cut into 2.5cm strips, and then half-moons

1 medium courgette, cut into 2.5cm pieces

1 medium red onion, cut into wedges

200g asparagus spears or tenderstem broccoli

For the marinade:

1 tablespoon olive oil

2 teaspoons lazy garlic

2 teaspoons fresh rosemary leaves, chopped (or 1 teaspoon dried rosemary)

Juice of 3 lemons, freshly squeezed

½ teaspoon sea salt

¼ teaspoon freshly ground black pepper

Mix all of the marinade ingredients together in a glass bowl. Add the chicken and coat thoroughly in the marinade. Pop the bowl into the fridge to chill for up to 6 hours.

Take the chicken out of the fridge and add the vegetables. Coat everything in the marinade and then thread the chicken, pepper, courgette and onion alternately on to four metal skewers.

Heat your grill. Cook the kebabs under a hot grill for 12–15 minutes, turning every few minutes.

For the last 5 minutes add the asparagus or broccoli to the grill and turn every minute until it is softened and slightly charred.

Once the chicken is no longer pink in the centre (cut open a piece to check), remove from the grill and serve with the asparagus or broccoli and a salad of your choice.

Lisa's tip: You can use wooden skewers for the kebabs instead of metal ones, but remember to soak them overnight

Per serving 138cals | 17g protein | 5g fat (1g saturates) | 6g carbs (5g total sugars) | 3g fibre

PORK MEDALLIONS
WITH ROASTED ROOT VEGETABLES

What a great alternative to a traditional Sunday roast. And, while you may not be having all the trimmings, you will be getting trimmer!

Serves 4

For the roasted vegetables:

3 carrots, peeled and cut into 1cm pieces

2 sweet potatoes, peeled and cut into 1cm pieces

1 onion, peeled and cut into 8 wedges

1 parsnip, peeled and cut into 2.5–5cm pieces

2 tablespoons olive oil

½ teaspoon dried rosemary

½ teaspoon dried thyme

1 teaspoon salt

1 teaspoon freshly ground black pepper

For the pork medallions:

500g pork tenderloin, trimmed and sliced into 2cm thick slices

2 teaspoons olive oil

Sea salt and freshly ground black pepper

Preheat the oven to 200°C/Fan 180°C/Gas 6.

Combine all the vegetables in a large roasting tin. Drizzle with the oil, rosemary, thyme, salt and pepper, and mix thoroughly.

Shake the vegetables into a single layer in the roasting tin and cook in the oven for 30–35 minutes, or until tender.

Take the slices of pork and, with the heel of your hand, press down to flatten them to half their thickness, then season with salt and pepper on both sides. Heat the oil in a heavy-bottomed pan on the hob over a medium-high heat. Sear the pork slices in the pan for around 3 minutes each side. You may need to do this in batches as you don't want to overcrowd the pan.

When the pork is nicely browned and cooked through, with no pink remaining, remove from the pan and serve with the roasted vegetables.

Per serving 409cals | 30g protein | 16g fat (4g saturates) | 32g carbs (14g total sugars) | 8g fibre

SESAME STEAK STIR-FRY

There are so many amazing flavours in this zesty stir-fry, and your other half is going to be so happy when you tell them you're cooking steak for dinner.

Serves 2

1 tablespoon sesame seeds

250g lean frying steak

2 tablespoons sesame oil

1 large red pepper, thinly sliced

125g green beans, trimmed

1 teaspoon lazy red chilli

1 large onion, sliced

1 tablespoon lazy garlic

1 tablespoon lazy ginger

2 tablespoons lime juice, freshly squeezed

2 tablespoons dark soy sauce

Sea salt and freshly ground black pepper

1 lime, quartered, to serve

In a hot frying pan toast the sesame seeds until golden brown. Move them around constantly in the pan so both sides are cooked. Set aside.

Trim any excess fat from the steak, and season with salt and pepper. Heat one tablespoon of the oil in a large frying pan on the hob over a medium-high heat. Add the steak and cook on each side for 3 minutes for medium, and up to 6 minutes for well done. Remove the steak from the pan and place on a chopping board to rest.

Add the remaining tablespoon of oil to the same pan, reduce the heat and gently sauté the pepper, green beans, chilli, onion, garlic and ginger for a few minutes until nearly tender. Add the lime juice and soy sauce and cook for a further 2–3 minutes.

Slice the steak into 1cm strips. Divide the vegetables between two plates and top with the sliced steak. Sprinkle with the toasted sesame seeds. Season and serve with the lime wedges.

Per serving 402cals | 31g protein | 23g fat (6g saturates) | 14g carbs (11g total sugars) | 6g fibre

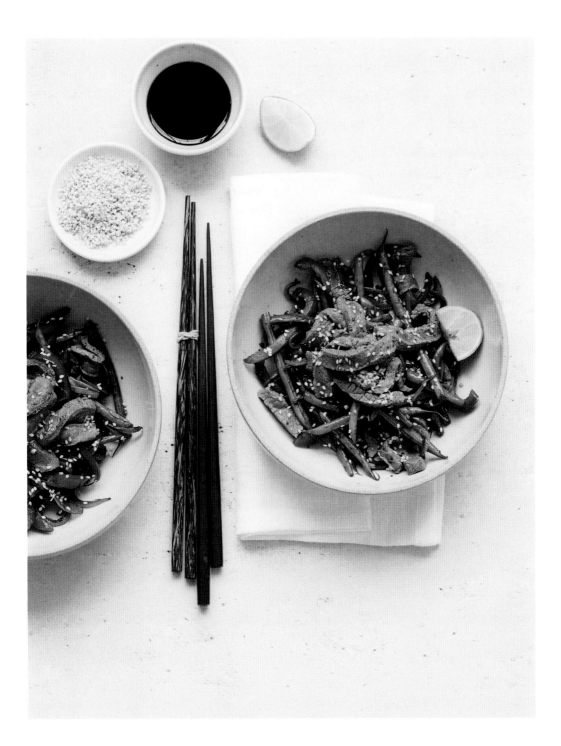

CHICKEN AND MUSHROOM POTS
WITH ROOT VEGETABLE MASH

This is a hearty, healthy take on chicken pie and mash. It tastes so good even my dad would happily have eaten it with no idea he was being virtuous.

Serves 4

250g carrots, diced
1 medium sweet potato
250g parsnips, diced
2 cloves of garlic, peeled
1 tablespoon olive oil
1 onion, thinly sliced
½ teaspoon fresh tarragon, finely chopped
100ml fresh chicken stock
295g tin condensed mushroom soup
300g cooked chicken, shredded
125g frozen peas
1 teaspoon wholegrain mustard
1 tablespoon semi-skimmed milk (optional)
Sea salt and freshly ground black pepper

Preheat the oven to 200°C/Fan 180°C/Gas 6.

Start by placing the carrots, sweet potato, parsnips and garlic cloves in a large saucepan. Cover with water and bring to the boil. Once boiling, cook the vegetables for around 15 minutes, or until tender.

While the vegetables are cooking, heat the oil in a large pan on the hob over a medium heat and sauté the onion for 5 minutes until translucent. Add the tarragon and chicken stock and increase the heat under the pan. Boil the stock until it has reduced by half.

Add the soup, chicken, frozen peas and mustard and simmer for 5 minutes. Divide between four ovenproof pie dishes. Cover with foil and bake in the oven for 10 minutes.

When the vegetables have softened, drain and mash them, adding salt and pepper and a tablespoon of semi-skimmed milk if you find the mash too dry.

Remove the pie dishes from the oven and serve on plates with the piping-hot root vegetable mash.

Per serving 329cals | 26g protein | 11g fat (2g saturates) | 27g carbs (11g total sugars) | 7g fibre

TURKEY MEATBALLS
WITH SWEET POTATO AND TOMATOES

This is great, filling family food. I often make it for my nephews because I know they love it. No spaghetti in sight!

Serves 2

1 large onion, chopped

1 teaspoon lazy garlic

Handful of fresh
  basil leaves

1 sprig of fresh thyme,
  leaves only

300g turkey mince

100g sweet potato,
  peeled and cut into
  1cm chunks

1 teaspoon olive oil

1 sprig of fresh
  rosemary, leaves only

10 cherry tomatoes

130g French beans

Sea salt and freshly
  ground black pepper

Preheat the oven to 180°C/Fan 160°C/Gas 4.

Put the onion, garlic, basil and thyme into a mini-chopper or food processor, and pulse everything into a rough paste.

Add this to the turkey mince and season with salt and pepper. Using your hands, mix everything well and massage it together until everything is well distributed. Shape the mixture into 10–12 small balls.

Line a baking tray with greaseproof paper and place the sweet potato on top. Add the coconut oil, sprinkle with the rosemary and toss everything together to make sure the sweet potato is well coated. Place into the preheated oven and cook for 10 minutes.

Remove the tray from the oven and stir the sweet potato to turn it and move it around. Place the meatballs on the same tray and return to the oven to cook for another 10 minutes. Add the cherry tomatoes to the tray and roast for a final 10 minutes.

Meanwhile, boil or steam the beans until tender, and serve everything together for a delicious balanced dinner.

Per serving 393cals | 46g protein | 13g fat (3g saturates) | 20g carbs (11g total sugars) | 6g fibre

CHICKEN AND ASPARAGUS TRAY BAKE

This is such a brilliant dish to whip up if you're hosting a dinner party, because it's so quick and simple to make but looks really impressive. It's also the kind of recipe you'll want to pass on to your friends.

Serves 4

4 boneless, skinless chicken breasts

1 tablespoon olive oil

2 lemons, sliced

2 x 250g asparagus bunches

Sea salt and freshly ground black pepper

1 tablespoon fresh flat-leaf parsley, chopped, to garnish

For the dressing:

Juice of 1 lemon, freshly squeezed

3 tablespoons clear honey

1 tablespoon lazy garlic

1 tablespoon fresh flat-leaf parsley, chopped

1 teaspoon sea salt

Freshly ground black pepper

Preheat the oven to 200°C/Fan 180°C/Gas 6.

Place the chicken breasts into a roasting tin and brush with a little olive oil. Season with salt and pepper.

To make the dressing, mix together the lemon juice, honey, garlic, parsley, salt and pepper. Pour three-quarters of the mixture over the chicken, keeping the rest for later on. Arrange three lemon slices on top of each chicken breast.

Bake the chicken for 15 minutes. Toss the asparagus in the remaining honey and lemon dressing. Take the roasting tin out of the oven and place the asparagus around the chicken. Season with salt and pepper. Return to the oven for 8–10 minutes or until the chicken is cooked through and the asparagus tender.

Serve with salad, and garnish with the chopped parsley.

Per serving 230cals | 31g protein | 6g fat (1g saturates) | 11g carbs (11g total sugars) | 3g fibre

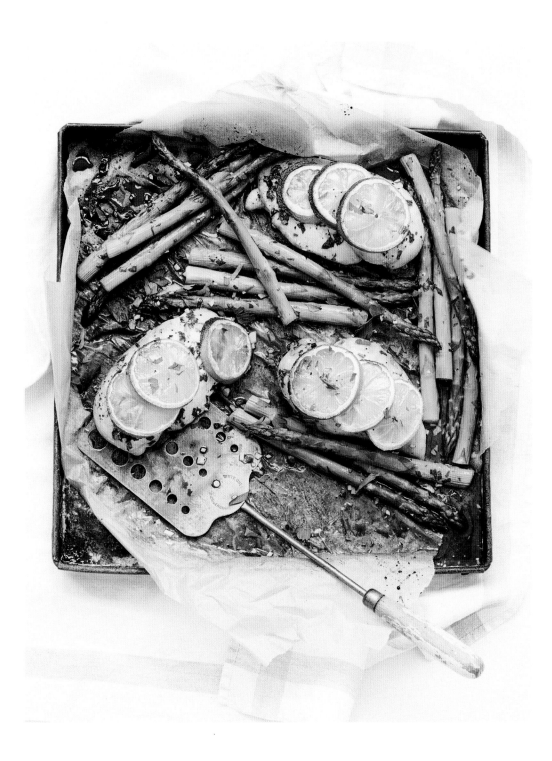

GRILLED SALMON
WITH BASIL, GARLIC AND WILTED SPINACH

This makes a brilliant lunch to have after you've done a morning gym class or training session, and it will fill you up for the rest of the day.

Serves 4

4 skinless salmon fillets
  (approximately 130g
  per fillet)
3 tablespoons water
450g bag fresh spinach
Sea salt and freshly ground
  black pepper
4 lemon wedges, to serve

For the dressing:

1 tablespoon olive oil
½ teaspoon lazy garlic
1 shallot, finely chopped
1 tablespoon fresh basil,
  finely chopped
1 tablespoon lemon juice,
  freshly squeezed
¼ teaspoon sea salt
¼ teaspoon freshly
  ground black pepper

Preheat the grill to a medium heat.

Heat the oil in a frying pan on the hob over a medium heat and sauté the garlic and shallot for 2 minutes. Next add the basil and lemon juice, followed by the salt and pepper. Cook, stirring continuously, for a further 2 minutes. Set aside.

Put the salmon fillets on to a baking tray, and season with salt and pepper.

Place the salmon under the grill and cook for 4 minutes. Turn the salmon and cook for another 4 minutes. Flip the salmon back over and pour a teaspoon of the garlic and basil dressing over each piece, making sure to cover the surface. Return to the grill for a final 2 minutes.

Place the water and spinach in a large saucepan on the hob over a low to medium heat. Cover and cook for about a minute until the spinach has wilted. Remove the lid and drain the water immediately, giving the spinach a squeeze with the back of a wooden spoon to remove as much as possible.

Divide the spinach between four plates. Add a salmon fillet and divide any remaining sauce. Serve with lemon wedges.

Per serving 342cals | 30g protein | 23g fat (4g saturates) | 2g carbs (2g total sugars) | 4g fibre

SPICY SEA BASS
WITH STEAMED VEGETABLES

Sea bass can be pricier than other fish, but it's very readily available so it's nice as a treat or if you're having friends over for dinner.

Serves 4

4 x 120g sea bass fillets, skin on, descaled

1 tablespoon coconut oil or olive oil

4 medium carrots, peeled and thinly sliced

1 head broccoli, cut into small florets

2 leeks, trimmed and thinly sliced

Sea salt and freshly ground black pepper

For the sauce:

1 tablespoon coconut oil

2 teaspoons lazy ginger

2 teaspoons lazy garlic

2 red chillies, deseeded and thinly sliced

4 spring onions, shredded lengthways

1 tablespoon soy sauce

Season the fish fillets with salt and pepper and then cut a few slashes into the skin side.

Add a tablespoon of oil to a frying pan on the hob and turn up the heat so that when you add the fish, skin side down, you hear it sizzle straight away. Press down on it gently to stop it curling.

Cook for 3–4 minutes and then turn it over and cook for another minute before transferring it to a warm serving plate. The skin should be slightly crispy.

Bring a large saucepan of salted water to the boil. Put the carrots into a steaming pan, or a bamboo steamer, and sit this on top of the pan of water. Cover and cook for 4 minutes. Add the broccoli and leeks to the carrots and cook for a further 4 minutes, or until they are to your preferred tenderness.

To make the sauce, heat the oil in a frying pan on the hob over a medium heat and sauté the ginger, garlic and chillies for 2 minutes. Add the spring onions and soy sauce and cook for a further 1 minute.

Serve the vegetables on a plate and lay a piece of the fish over the top with some of the sauce spooned over.

Per serving 344cals | 29g protein | 18g fat (8g saturates) | 11g carbs (9g total sugars) | 9g fibre

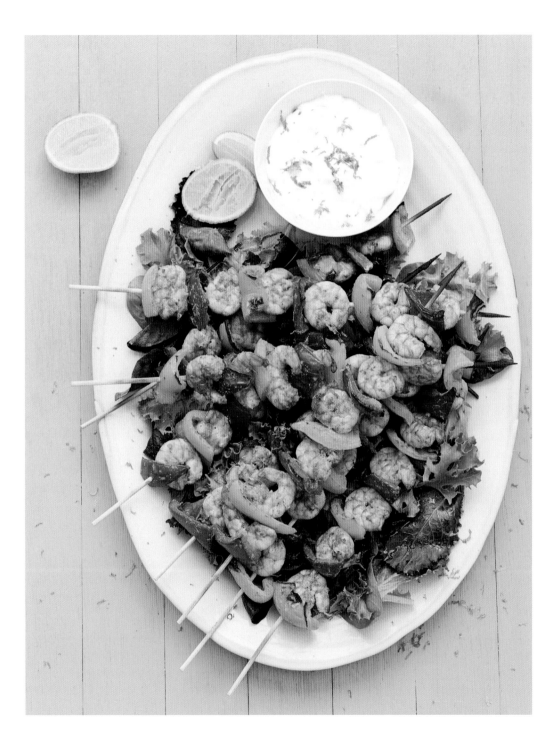

PRAWN KEBABS
WITH LIME YOGHURT

This is the sort of dish I tend to eat when I go out. It's a great barbecue go-to, so you don't have to feel like you're missing out at summer get-togethers when everyone else is tucking into the hot dogs.

Serves 2

1 red pepper

1 yellow pepper

2 tablespoons curry powder

1 teaspoon lazy garlic

1 tablespoon coconut oil or olive oil

1 tablespoon lemon juice, freshly squeezed

Juice and zest of half a lime

300g shelled fresh king prawns

3 tablespoons low-fat Greek yoghurt

Sea salt and freshly ground black pepper

Salad leaves, to serve

Chop both the peppers into 2.5cm chunks. In a bowl combine the curry powder, garlic, oil, lemon and lime juice. Season well. Add the prawns to the bowl and mix together with the peppers so they are well coated with the mixture.

Slide the prawns on to wooden skewers, putting a pepper chunk between each one. Place the skewers under the grill and cook for 8 minutes, turning every 2 minutes.

While the prawns are cooking, mix together the yoghurt and lime zest. Place the skewers on top of a large green salad and drizzle with the lime yoghurt.

Lisa's tip: When using wooden skewers, remember to soak them overnight.

Per serving 303cals | 37g protein | 10g fat (6g saturates) | 13g carbs (9g total sugars) | 8g fibre

GARLIC AND CHILLI PRAWNS

This punchy recipe has quite full-on flavours, and that's the way I like it. But if you're not a fan of either garlic or chilli, there's no law that says you have to use both! Feel free to experiment.

Serves 4

2 tablespoons olive oil

3 garlic cloves, thinly sliced

3 red chillies, thinly sliced

1 medium tomato, deseeded and finely chopped

2 tablespoons fresh flat-leaf parsley, chopped

400g king prawns, raw

140g bag mixed salad leaves

1 avocado, cut into chunks

10 cherry tomatoes, halved

Lemon wedges, to serve

Heat the oil in a large frying pan on the hob over a medium-high heat. Add the garlic and chilli, and cook for 1 minute until fragrant. Stir in the tomato and parsley.

Add the prawns and cook for 2–3 minutes, stirring occasionally, until the prawns are pink.

Remove from the heat and serve with the salad leaves, avocado and tomatoes. Garnish with the lemon wedges.

Per serving 243cals | 20g protein | 16g fat (3g saturates) | 3g carbs (3g total sugars) | 4g fibre

LEMON PRAWNS

Prawns can be cooked in so many different ways, and you don't have to be a super chef to get them right. The sharpness of the lemon in this recipe gives your mouth a real wake-up call.

Serves 4

400g shelled fresh king
  prawns
1 red onion, finely diced
Quarter of a stick of
  celery, finely diced
1 tablespoon fresh flat-leaf
  parsley, finely chopped
140g bag mixed
  salad leaves
Half a cucumber, sliced
12 cherry tomatoes, halved

For the dressing:

2 tablespoons olive oil
Juice of 2 lemons,
  freshly squeezed
½ teaspoon clear honey
½ teaspoon sea salt
½ teaspoon freshly ground
  black pepper

In a large bowl mix the prawns, onion, celery and parsley.

To make the dressing, whisk together the oil, lemon juice, honey, salt and pepper until they are thoroughly mixed.

Pour the dressing over the prawn mixture, and toss to combine. Serve on a bed of salad leaves, cucumber and tomatoes.

Per serving 163cals | 19g protein | 7g fat (1g saturates) | 6g carbs (5g total sugars) | 2g fibre

MIXED SEAFOOD LETTUCE CUPS

These seafood cups look so pretty. Popping the mixture in lettuce leaves makes a brilliant healthy alternative to bread or pastry. They're lovely to serve up if you've got mates coming round.

Serves 4

3 tablespoons light mayonnaise

1 tablespoon fresh dill, chopped

1 tablespoon lemon juice, freshly squeezed

150g small prawns

120g crab meat, fresh or tinned

120g tin tuna in spring water

8 cherry tomatoes, halved

8 cos lettuce leaves

Extra dill fronds, to garnish

In a bowl, mix together the mayonnaise, dill and lemon juice. Add the prawns, crab, tuna and tomatoes, and mix gently.

Lay out the lettuce leaves and fill each one with the seafood mixture. Top with a few extra dill fronds and serve immediately.

Per serving 145cals | 19g protein | 6g fat (1g saturates) | 3g carbs (2g total sugars) | 1g fibre

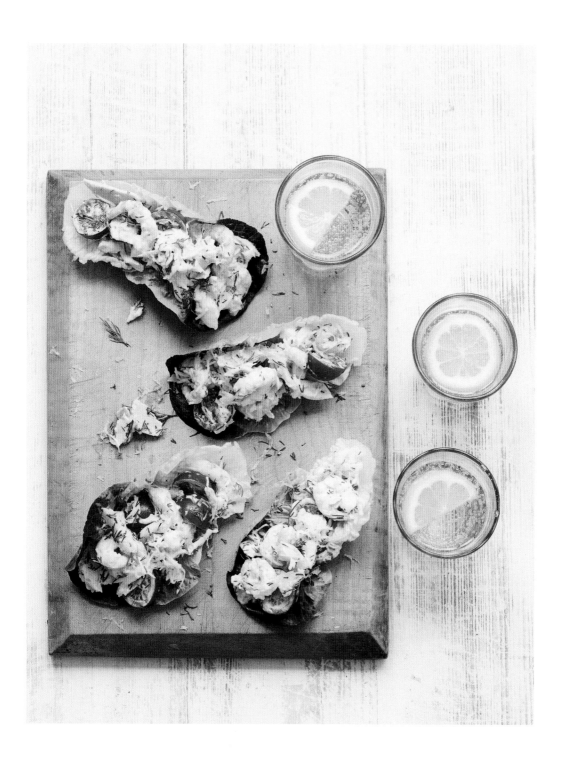

SOY SCALLOP AND PRAWN STIR-FRY

Don't fear scallops! I used to be intimidated by them, but now I couldn't be without them in my life. They're so versatile and quick to cook, and easy to buy in the supermarket from the fish counter or fish aisle.

Serves 4

2 tablespoons soy sauce
½ teaspoon ground ginger
1 tablespoon olive oil
350g small broccoli florets
1 red chilli, sliced
1 large sweet red pepper, deseeded, cut into strips
2 teaspoons lazy ginger
1 teaspoon lazy garlic
150g button mushrooms, stemmed and cut in half
12 scallops
360g large prawns, raw

In a bowl, mix the soy sauce and ground ginger together. Set aside.

Heat the oil in a large wok or sauté pan and stir-fry the broccoli, chilli and sweet pepper for 3–4 minutes on a high heat, stirring all the time.

Add the lazy ginger and garlic and stir-fry for around 30 seconds until fragrant.

Add the mushrooms, scallops, prawns and soy sauce mixture. Reduce the heat to medium and cook for 4–5 minutes, stirring continuously, until the scallops are cooked through and the prawns have turned pink. Serve immediately.

Per serving 231cals | 39g protein | 5g fat (1g saturates) | 6g carbs (5g total sugars) | 5g fibre

GINGER, CHILLI AND LEMON SALMON

Ginger isn't for everyone, and it took me a while to embrace it. But it's so good for you. Not only does it aid digestion, it also improves your circulation and even helps with pain relief. I often include it in smoothies, and I even eat it raw now and then.

Serves 2

2 medium-sized salmon
  steaks (approximately
  130g per steak)
1 teaspoon olive oil

For the dressing:

1 red chilli, sliced
½ teaspoon lazy garlic
½ tablespoon lazy ginger
1 tablespoon lemon juice,
  freshly squeezed
2 teaspoons sesame oil
2 teaspoons soy sauce

Preheat the oven to 180°C/Fan 160°C/Gas 4.

Put all of the dressing ingredients into a jar, put the lid on and shake well.

Lay the salmon steaks on to separate pieces of tin foil. Brush each steak with a little oil and top with the dressing.

Fold in the foil to make sealed parcels and place on to a baking tray. Cook in the oven for 10–12 minutes.

Once cooked, unwrap each parcel carefully and serve the fish with a side salad, using the juices from the fish parcels as a flavoursome dressing.

Per serving 327cals | 27g protein | 24g fat (4g saturates) | 1g carbs (1g total sugars) | 0g fibre

PORTOBELLO MUSHROOM 'PIZZAS'

Dough is a definite no-no. But thanks to these magic 'pizzas', you'll still feel like you're indulging when you have a cosy family movie night in.

Serves 2

2 large field mushrooms
10 basil leaves, finely chopped
8 cherry tomatoes, sliced
100g soft goat's cheese
Sea salt and freshly ground black pepper
80g rocket, to serve

Preheat the oven to 180°C/Fan 160°C/Gas 4.

Remove the stalks of the mushrooms. With a piece of kitchen paper brush them clean. Line a baking tray with foil and scrunch it into shape so that it will support the mushrooms when they are full of filling. Place the mushrooms stalk side up. Add a few basil leaves around the top of the mushrooms, followed by a layer of the tomatoes.

Crumble the goat's cheese over the top, covering the herbs and tomatoes evenly. Add another layer of basil and tomatoes, then season with salt and pepper.

Bake in the oven for 10–15 minutes. Keep an eye on it to make sure the cheese doesn't burn. Remove from the oven, and serve on a bed of rocket.

Per serving 190cals | 14g protein | 14g fat (9g saturates) | 3g carbs (3g total sugars) | 2g fibre

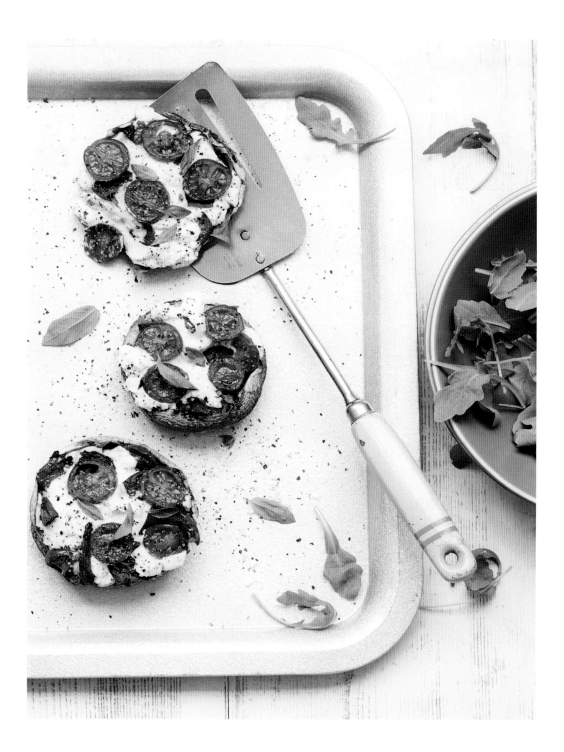

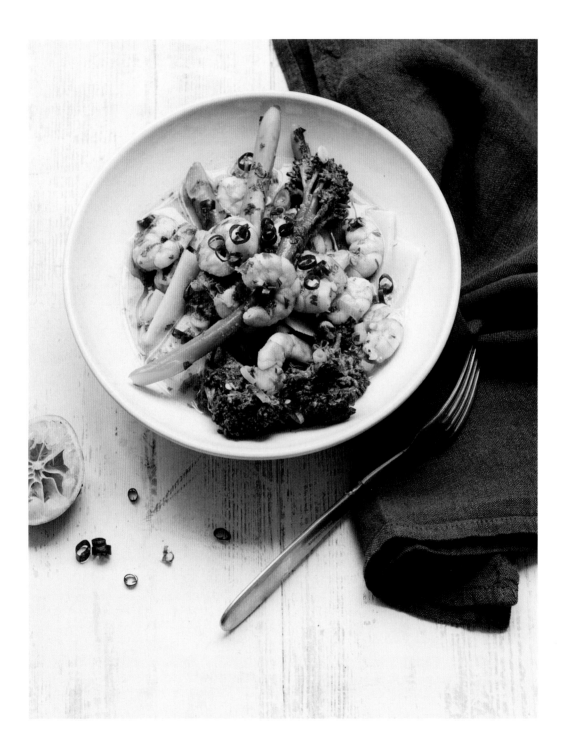

THAI GREEN PRAWN AND BROCCOLI CURRY

This is an amazing taste of South-East Asia, but please don't treat it like a soup. You should definitely be eating more of the prawns and veg than the sauce, tempting as it is.

Serves 4

400ml tin low-fat coconut milk

2 tablespoons Thai green curry paste

5ml fish sauce

1 teaspoon clear honey

200g tenderstem broccoli

5 spring onions, finely sliced

400g fresh tiger prawns, raw

225g tin sliced bamboo shoots, drained

Zest and juice of 1 lime

4 tablespoons fresh coriander leaves, chopped

½ teaspoon dried chilli or chilli flakes, to serve

Pour the coconut milk, curry paste, fish sauce and honey into a large pan. Slowly bring to the boil on the hob over a low-to-medium heat. Add the broccoli and reduce the heat. Cover and simmer for 4 minutes, or until tender.

Stir in the spring onions, prawns and bamboo shoots. Bring back to the boil and simmer, stirring occasionally. When the prawns have turned pink, after around 3–4 minutes, stir in the lime zest and juice, as well as the coriander leaves.

Divide into four bowls and top with some of the dried chilli or chilli flakes.

Per serving 214cals | 22g protein | 11g fat (7g saturates) | 6g carbs (4g total sugars) | 4g fibre

BAKED AVOCADO
WITH HAM AND EGGS

I'd only ever had avocados cold in salads, so for a long time I had no idea how amazing they taste when they're warm. This meal looks really impressive, with the eggs baked in the avocado hollows, but it's also really very quick and easy to make.

Serves 2

1 avocado, cut in half
  with the stone removed

2 small eggs

4 small thyme sprigs,
  leaves picked

2 slices ham

Sea salt and freshly ground
  black pepper

Preheat the oven to 200°C/Fan 180°C/Gas 6.

Place the avocado halves on to a baking tray. Carefully scoop out a little more of the avocado to make a slightly bigger hole that will fit as much egg as possible. Crack the eggs into the holes. Season with the fresh thyme leaves and a little salt and pepper.

Gently place the baking dish in the oven and bake for around 12–15 minutes, until the eggs are cooked. Serve with the ham on the side.

Per serving 286cals | 12g protein | 25g fat (6g saturates) | 2g carbs (1g total sugars) | 5g fibre

BAKED AUBERGINE
WITH TOMATO AND HALLOUMI

I'll be honest, I was always a bit suspicious of aubergines, but now I use them in dishes all the time. I consider baked aubergines to be a good alternative to baked potatoes.

Serves 4

2 medium aubergines, sliced into 1cm rounds

1 tablespoon olive oil

1 large onion, finely chopped

3 teaspoons lazy garlic

2 x 400g tins chopped tomatoes

1 tablespoon dried basil

1 tablespoon dried thyme

1 tablespoon dried oregano

30g fresh flat-leaf parsley, finely chopped

20 black olives, cut in half

250g block halloumi cheese, cut into 5mm slices

10g Parmesan, grated

Sea salt and freshly ground black pepper

Preheat the oven to 200°C/Fan 180°C/Gas 6.

Lay out the aubergines in a single layer on a lined baking tray (or two if you need to). Brush a little oil on to the top of each slice. Roast in the oven for 10 minutes on each side. Remove the tray from the oven and flip the slices over. Brush with a little more oil and bake for another 10 minutes. Remove from the oven and reduce the heat to 190°C/Fan 170°C/Gas 5.

Heat the remaining oil in a frying pan on the hob over a medium heat. Sauté the onion for 5 minutes until translucent. Add the garlic and stir for another 30 seconds or so. Mix in the tomatoes, herbs and olives, and simmer for another 5–10 minutes, or until the sauce has thickened slightly. Season to taste.

Pour a third of the tomato sauce into an ovenproof dish. Place a layer of the aubergines on top of that, followed by a layer of the halloumi slices. Repeat to make a second layer. Finish with the final third of the tomato sauce, and top with grated Parmesan.

Place the dish in the oven for 20 minutes until it is bubbling and the cheese is golden. Remove and enjoy!

Per serving 332cals | 20g protein | 20g fat (12g saturates) | 14g carbs (13g total sugars) | 7g fibre

SWEETCORN FRITTERS
WITH HERBED YOGHURT

Fritter' is a word that conjures up fatty, unhealthy images of fried food, but you really can eat these without feeling guilty. And they taste so good.

Serves 4

220ml low-fat natural yoghurt
25g fresh chives, chopped
325g tin sweetcorn
240g tin cannellini beans, drained
160g polenta
40g wholemeal flour
60ml semi-skimmed milk
1 egg
1 tablespoon cayenne pepper
Olive oil, for frying
Sea salt and freshly ground black pepper
Salad leaves, to serve

Combine the yoghurt and chives in a small bowl and mix thoroughly. Place in the fridge to keep cool.

Place the sweetcorn and beans into a food processor along with the polenta, flour, milk, egg, cayenne pepper and seasoning. Pulse a few times to mix and break everything down so the ingredients have a rough consistency. Transfer to a mixing bowl and stir until well combined. Allow the mixture to stand for 10 minutes.

Once the 10 minutes are up, heat a little oil in a frying pan on the hob over a medium heat. Drop a tangerine-sized amount of the sweetcorn mixture into the frying pan and flatten out into a fritter. Cook until golden brown on both sides (approximately 2–3 minutes each side). Repeat until all the fritters are cooked.

Serve immediately with the herbed yoghurt and a fresh green salad.

Per serving 373cals | 14g protein | 10g fat (2g saturates) | 53g carbs (9g total sugars) | 7g fibre

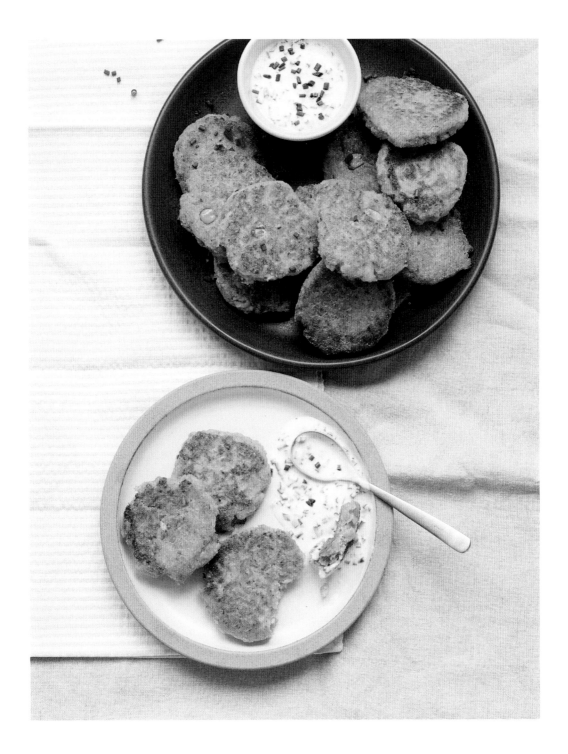

GARLIC AND CHILLI COD
WITH ROASTED SPINACH AND CAULIFLOWER

This is one of those easy, brilliant, 'bung it all in the oven' recipes that I love. Full of flavour, it's very satisfying, too.

Serves 2

Half a cauliflower head, cut into florets

250g spinach, washed

½ teaspoon smoked paprika

1 teaspoon lazy garlic

½ tablespoon olive oil

Juice of half a lemon, freshly squeezed

2 x 150g cod fillets, with the skin on

1 tablespoon harissa paste

Sea salt and freshly ground black pepper

1 tablespoon fresh chives, chopped, to garnish

For the salsa:

150g cherry tomatoes, quartered

Juice of half a lime, freshly squeezed

1 teaspoon lazy chilli

½ tablespoon olive oil

1 tablespoon fresh chives, chopped

Preheat the oven to 200°C/Fan 180°C/Gas 6.

Put the cauliflower florets and spinach in an ovenproof dish. Sprinkle the paprika, garlic, oil and lemon juice over the vegetables and mix well with your hands. Season with salt and pepper and cook on the top shelf of the oven for 10 minutes.

Meanwhile, season the cod with salt and pepper and rub in the harissa paste. Place on a foil-lined baking tray.

Once the vegetables have been in the oven for the first 10 minutes, turn the oven down to 180°C/Fan 160°C/Gas 4, pop the fish on to the centre shelf of the oven and cook for 10–12 minutes.

To create the salsa, mix the tomatoes with the lime juice, chilli, oil and chives.

Serve the vegetables topped with the fish and salsa, and sprinkle over the chives to garnish.

Per serving 261cals | 33g protein | 8g fat (1g saturates) | 10g carbs (8g total sugars) | 7g fibre

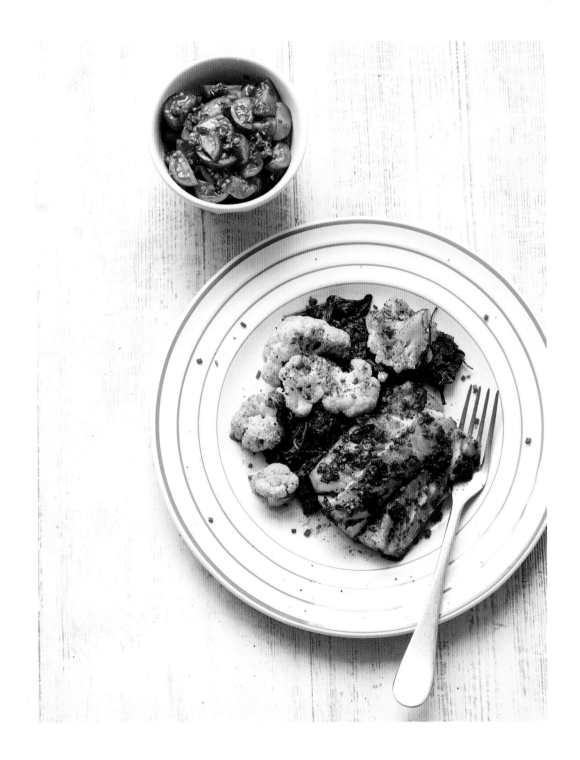

BAKED HAKE
WITH CRUSHED PEAS AND GARLIC CAULIFLOWER

This dish is your healthy alternative to fried fish and mushy peas. It's filling beyond words, and the sweetness of the peas contrasts so nicely with the savoury flavour of the cauliflower.

Serves 4

1 large cauliflower, cut into small florets

4 tablespoons olive oil

4 cloves garlic, peeled and crushed

4 x 150g hake fillets

1 lemon, sliced

250g frozen peas

1 tablespoon lemon juice, freshly squeezed

20g fresh flat-leaf parsley, chopped

Sea salt and freshly ground black pepper

Preheat the oven to190°C/Fan 170°C/Gas 5.

In a large roasting tin, mix together the cauliflower florets, 2 tablespoons of the olive oil and the garlic. Season with salt and pepper and spread out evenly. Cook in the oven for 15 minutes.

Line a large ovenproof dish with tin foil. Lay the fish on the foil, skin side down, and drizzle with the remaining olive oil. Place the lemon slices around the side, and season well.

After the first 15 minutes, stir the cauliflower. Return the roasting tray to the oven along with the fish for 8–10 minutes, until it is flaky and cooked through.

Meanwhile, place the peas into a pan of boiling salted water and cook for 4–5 minutes. Drain and return to the pan. Add the lemon juice, and a pinch of salt and pepper to taste. Use a potato masher to crush the peas so they have a rough texture.

Divide between four plates, and sprinkle with the fresh parsley.

Per serving 331cals | 34g protein | 15g fat (2g saturates) | 12g carbs (7g total sugars) | 6g fibre

ROASTED MONKFISH
WITH GARLIC, ROSEMARY AND PUY LENTILS

Monkfish is super tasty and really meaty. It will fill a plate and your tummy. Puy lentils can also be bought ready cooked, in pouches, if you don't have time to cook from scratch.

Serves 2

150g puy lentils

2 x 120g monkfish tails (skinless and sinew removed)

1 clove of fresh garlic, thinly sliced

1 tablespoon olive oil

3 sprigs of fresh rosemary

Sea salt and freshly ground black pepper

1 lemon, cut into wedges, to serve

Large handful of fresh flat-leaf parsley, finely chopped

Preheat the oven to 200°C/Fan 180°C/Gas 6.

Rinse the lentils under cold running water and then place in a large pan of water. Bring to the boil on the hob over a medium heat. Once they begin to simmer, reduce the heat slightly and cook the lentils for 25 minutes, or until they are tender. Drain, season to taste and stir well.

While the lentils are cooking, slash the monkfish in sections diagonally across the body at 2cm intervals and insert slices of garlic. Season well with salt and pepper.

Lightly oil a roasting tin. Lay the rosemary sprigs in the tin and top with the fish. Roast for 10–12 minutes until the fish is cooked through.

Serve the monkish on a bed of the lentils. Squeeze over some lemon juice and sprinkle with chopped parsley.

Per serving 372cals | 37g protein | 7g fat (1g saturates) | 35g carbs (1g total sugars) | 9g fibre

TUNA STEAK
WITH ROASTED VEGETABLES

I eat this dish for lunch all the time when I'm filming. It's fuss free, super healthy and so delicious. Tuna is a great option in restaurants, too, as it's usually cooked and served quite healthily, like this.

Serves 2

2 large carrots, sliced on the diagonal
2 courgettes, sliced on the diagonal
3 teaspoons lazy garlic
3 tablespoons olive oil
Juice and zest of 1 lemon
2 x 120g tuna steaks
8 asparagus spears
Sea salt and freshly ground black pepper
Lemon wedges, to serve

Preheat the oven to 200°C/Fan 180°C/Gas 6.

Toss the carrots, courgettes and garlic in 1½ tablespoons of oil, and season with salt and pepper. Place in an ovenproof dish and cook for around 15 minutes.

For a quick marinade, rub the lemon juice and some pepper into both sides of the tuna and leave for 5 minutes. Reserve the lemon zest for later on.

After the first 15 minutes, stir the vegetables. Add the asparagus spears and another ½ tablespoon of olive oil. Place back in the oven for another 8–10 minutes.

Season the tuna steaks with salt. Heat the remaining tablespoon of oil in a frying pan on the hob over a medium heat. Cook the steaks on one side until the bottom third of each is brown, and then flip them over with a spatula and cook the other side for the same amount of time. The middle should remain pink – unless you like your fish well done, in which case continue cooking until the whole of the fish turns brown.

Divide the roasted vegetables between two bowls and top each with a tuna steak. Sprinkle the lemon zest over the fish and serve immediately with lemon wedges.

Per serving 352cals | 34g protein | 18g fat (3g saturates) | 10g carbs (9g total sugars) | 6g fibre

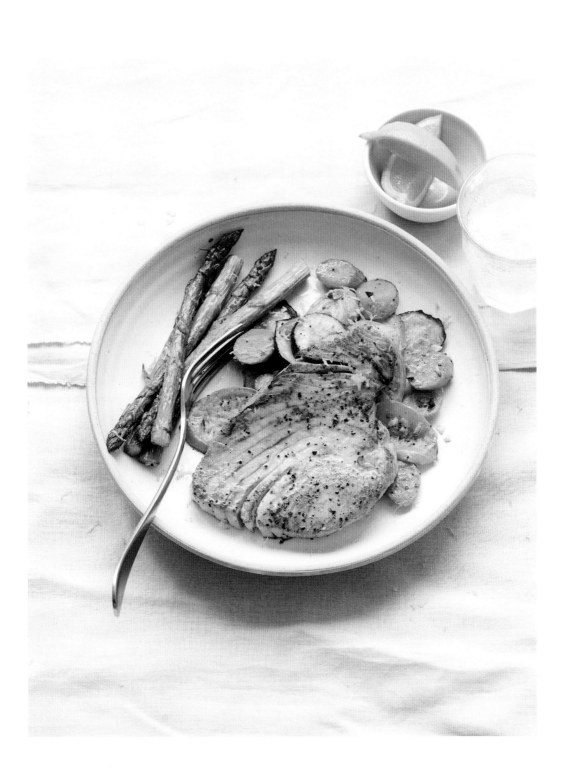

FRUITY COUSCOUS
WITH BOILED EGG AND ROASTED VEGETABLES

These may not be the most obvious ingredients to put together, but, take it from me, this recipe works. It's ideal for a lunchbox, or food on the run.

Serves 4

1 red pepper, sliced into strips

1 green pepper, sliced into strips

1 courgette, sliced

2 tablespoons olive oil

1 large white onion, finely chopped

1 tablespoon lazy garlic

1 tablespoon lemon juice, freshly squeezed

250g cooked chicken breast, chopped into 1cm chunks

100g couscous

2 tablespoons sultanas, roughly chopped

1 tablespoon flaked coconut

175ml fresh chicken stock

2 tablespoons fresh coriander leaves, finely chopped

2 hard-boiled eggs, cut into quarters

Sea salt and freshly ground black pepper

Lemon wedges, to serve

Preheat the oven to 180°C/Fan 160°C/Gas 4.

Mix the peppers and courgette in a bowl with 1 tablespoon of the olive oil, and season with salt and pepper. Lay the vegetables out on a non-stick baking tray and roast in the oven for 30 minutes.

Heat the remaining oil in a saucepan on the hob over a medium heat. Sauté the onion, garlic and lemon juice for 2 minutes. Add the chicken and the roasted vegetables, and stir to make sure they are well coated.

Put the couscous, sultanas and coconut flakes in a mixing bowl.

Heat the chicken stock gently in a pan on the hob over a low to medium heat. Bring it to the boil, then remove from the heat and pour over the couscous. Cover with cling film and leave to stand for a few minutes, or until all the stock is absorbed and the couscous is tender.

Fluff the couscous with a fork. Add the chicken, roasted vegetables and coriander. Mix together well.

Lay the egg quarters on top and serve with fresh lemon wedges on the side.

Per serving 356cals | 23g protein | 12g fat (4g saturates) | 36g carbs (16g total sugars) | 4g fibre

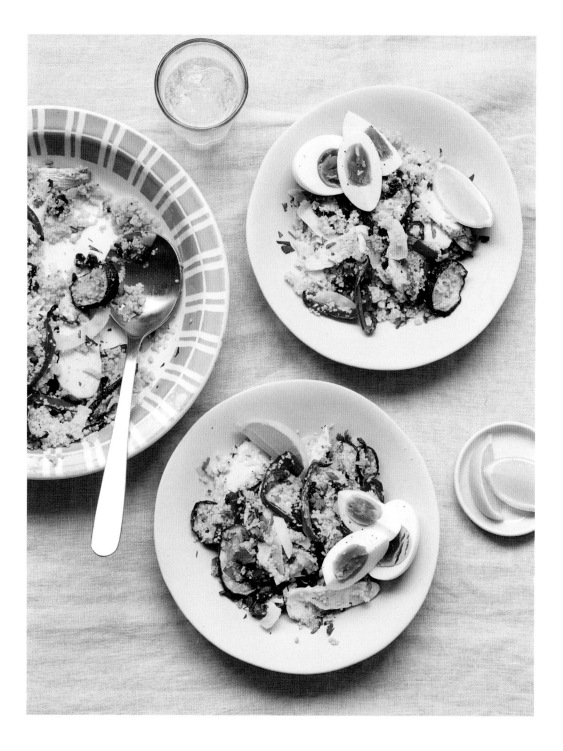

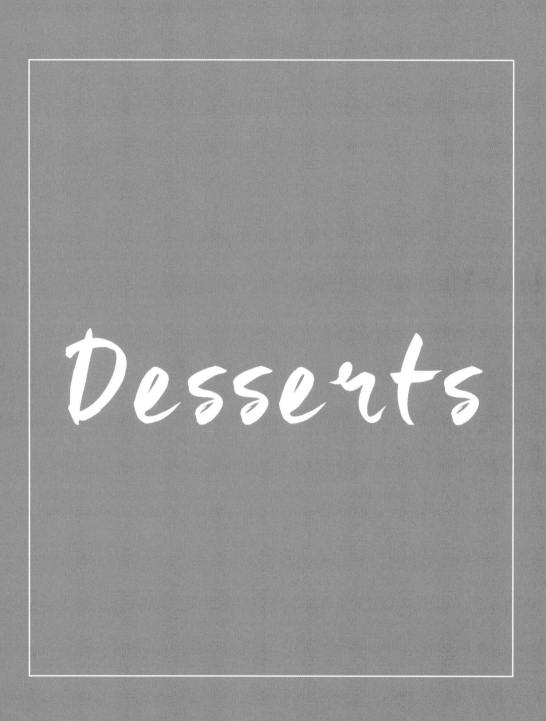

Desserts

FRUITY ICE TREATS

You can enjoy these icy treats with children, and they'll love helping you make them. Why not pop the citrus ice cubes in a big glass of still or sparkling water to liven it up as a virtuous alternative to squash or juice?

Serves 2 or more

For the citrus cubes:

Juice of 1 lemon,
  freshly squeezed
Juice of 1 lime,
  freshly squeezed
Juice of 1 orange,
  freshly squeezed

For the raspberry and
pomegranate ice lollies:

150g raspberries, fresh
  or frozen
50g pomegranate seeds
2 tablespoons low-fat
  yoghurt (optional)

To make the citrus cubes, simply mix the fresh juice of a whole lemon, lime and orange. Pour into ice cube trays and pop into the freezer for 2–3 hours.

For the ice lollies, pop the raspberries and pomegranate into a blender and whizz until smooth. Pour into two ice-lolly moulds and ideally freeze overnight, but a minimum of 5 hours until set.

Lisa's tip: For a creamier version of the ice lollies, you can add some low-fat yoghurt to the fruit.

Per serving (cubes) 12cals | 0g protein, 0g fat (0g saturates) | 3g carbs (3g total sugars) | 0g fibre

Per serving (per lolly) 78cals | 4g protein | 1g fat (0g saturates) | 12g carbs (10g total sugars) | 4g fibre

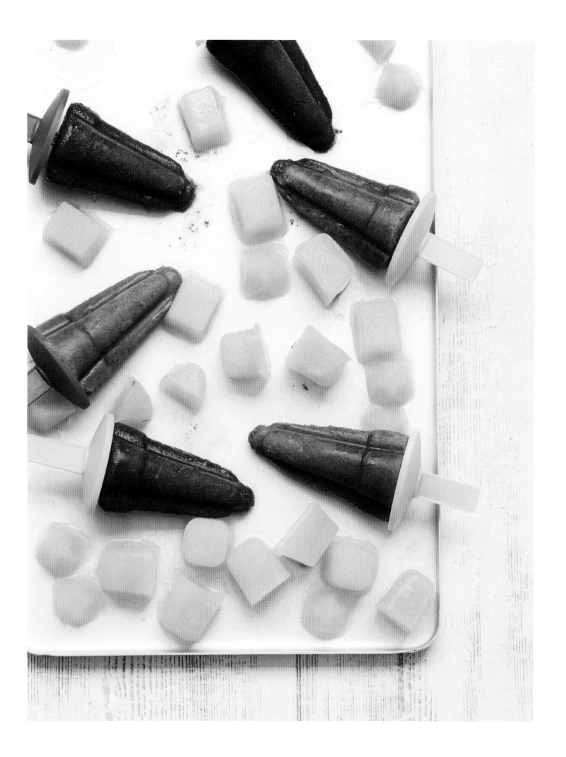

FROZEN YOGHURT

If you look on the back of a pot of frozen yoghurt you'll be shocked at what it contains, especially when you can make this incredible version yourself with so few ingredients.

Serves 4

400g frozen blueberries
  or mango
120g low-fat Greek yoghurt
2 teaspoons vanilla extract
3 tablespoons clear honey

Place all the ingredients into the bowl of a food processor. Blend until totally smooth. If the mixture seems a bit thick to blitz, wait a few minutes for the berries to defrost slightly so that the juice helps the fruit to blend.

Transfer the yoghurt to an airtight container, and freeze.

Lisa's tip: This delicious yoghurt should keep for around 3–4 weeks in the freezer.

Per serving 98cals | 4g protein | 1g fat (0g saturates) | 18g carbs (18g total sugars) | 2g fibre

BANANA OAT COOKIES

This is the biscuit you're allowed. But please remember that they're not for elevenses or a three o'clock snack. We're not hamsters, and we don't need to nibble constantly. These are strictly to eat at the end of mealtimes only.

Makes approximately 16 cookies

4 ripe bananas, mashed
60ml almond or oat milk
1 teaspoon ground cinnamon
320g porridge oats

Preheat the oven to 180°C/Fan 160°C/Gas 4.

Mix together the bananas, milk, cinnamon and porridge oats.

Line a baking sheet with non-stick baking parchment. Drop tablespoonfuls of the mixture on to the baking sheet and flatten down with the back of a spoon until they are 5–6cm wide and 1cm thick.

Bake in the oven for 25–30 minutes until golden brown.

Per serving 107cals | 3g protein | 2g fat (0g saturates) | 19g carbs (5g total sugars) | 2g fibre

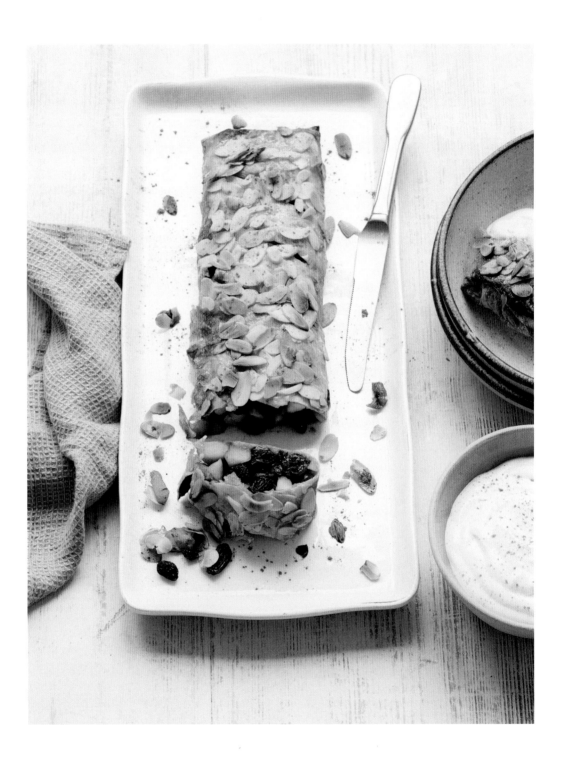

APPLE AND CINNAMON STRUDEL

It's best to make this to share with family and friends, and your slice needs to be small! If the strudel doesn't all get eaten and you're worried you're going to pick at the leftovers, pop it in the freezer and only ever defrost a little bit at a time. Think twice: don't go for the extra slice.

Serves 4

300g Golden Delicious apples, diced

100g sultanas

½ teaspoon ground cinnamon

1 tablespoon clear honey

3 sheets of filo pastry

1 egg white, lightly beaten

25g flaked almonds

2 teaspoons low-fat crème fraîche (optional), to serve

Extra cinnamon (optional), to garnish

Preheat the oven to 190°C/Fan 170°C/Gas 5.

Cook the apples, sultanas, cinnamon and three-quarters of a tablespoon of honey in a saucepan on the hob over a low heat for 8–10 minutes, or until the fruit is soft.

When you are ready to assemble the strudel, unroll the filo pastry sheets. Brush one sheet with egg white, place another sheet on top of it, and repeat twice. Spoon the fruit mixture lengthways across one edge of the pastry, leaving 1cm of space at each end. Roll up the strudel, beginning with the side where the filling is and working across to the other side so you are left with a long tube shape. Press the edges together firmly to seal, and seal the ends well with egg white.

Line a baking tray with greaseproof paper and carefully place the strudel on to the tray. Brush the remaining honey across the top and slash the pastry at 2cm intervals along the length of the strudel. Scatter over the flaked almonds and bake in the oven for 30–40 minutes.

Allow the strudel to cool for 5 minutes, and serve with a little low-fat crème fraîche. Sprinkle with extra cinnamon if required.

Lisa's tip: Filo pastry sheets can dry out very quickly, so keep them wrapped or covered until you're ready to use them.

Per serving (including crème fraiche) 255cals | 6g protein | 6g fat (1g saturates) | 44g carbs (28g total sugars) | 3g fibre

STRAWBERRY CARPACCIO
WITH PISTACHIOS, YOGHURT AND CINNAMON

Old Lisa was the queen of trifle, but this is my new, improved, vastly healthier version of it. You've still got the amazing layers of fruity flavour, but without all the extra sugar and additives.

Serves 4

400g strawberries, hulled and thinly sliced

2 tablespoons ground cinnamon

200g low-fat yoghurt

A little honey, for drizzling

30g pistachios, roughly chopped, to garnish

Arrange the strawberries in a thin layer over a large plate or platter.

Mix the cinnamon into the yoghurt and set aside.

Drizzle some honey over the strawberries, and scatter the pistachios to garnish the fruit.

Serve with the cinnamon yoghurt.

Per serving (without honey) 114cals | 5g protein | 5g fat (1g saturates) | 10g carbs (10g total sugars) | 4g fibre

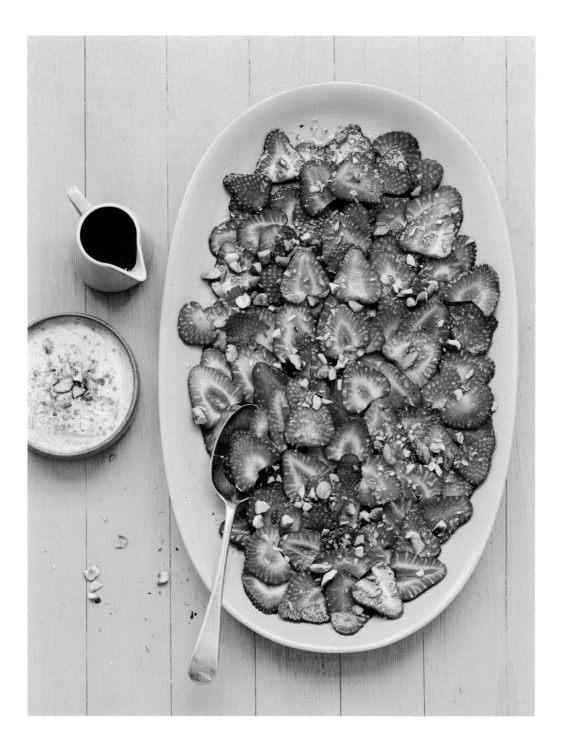

GRANOLA BARS

I am a massive fan of granola, and these bars are great breakfast and handbag food. They're not something you should be snacking on often, but they'll be your saviour if you feel like you're about to reach for crisps or chocolate.

Makes 12 bars

340g rolled oats
40g dried cherries
40g dried apricots
40g raisins
120g sliced almonds
2 tablespoons wheatgerm
¼ teaspoon salt
1 large egg
2 large egg whites
100ml clear honey
½ teaspoon vanilla extract

Preheat the oven to 160°C/Fan 140°C/Gas 3.

Whizz 80g of the oats in a blender until they resemble coarse flour. Set aside.

Put the dried fruit into a food processor, and pulse until coarsely chopped. Combine the remaining oats, oat flour, almonds, wheatgerm and salt in a bowl, then add the chopped dried fruit.

In another bowl, whisk the egg and the egg whites lightly using a fork. Add the honey and the vanilla, and mix well. Pour the wet mixture into the dry oat mixture and use a fork to combine them until everything is well covered with the egg mix.

Line a 25cm x 30cm rectangular lipped baking tray with greaseproof paper. Spoon the granola mixture into the pan and press firmly, making sure it's even and flat. Bake in the oven for 20 minutes until lightly browned.

Turn out on to a cooling rack. Once the granola reaches room temperature, cut into 12 slices.

Lisa's tip: These tasty bars can be stored in an airtight container for up to a week.

Per serving 249cals | 8g protein | 9g fat (1g saturates) | 33g carbs (13g total sugars) | 3g fibre

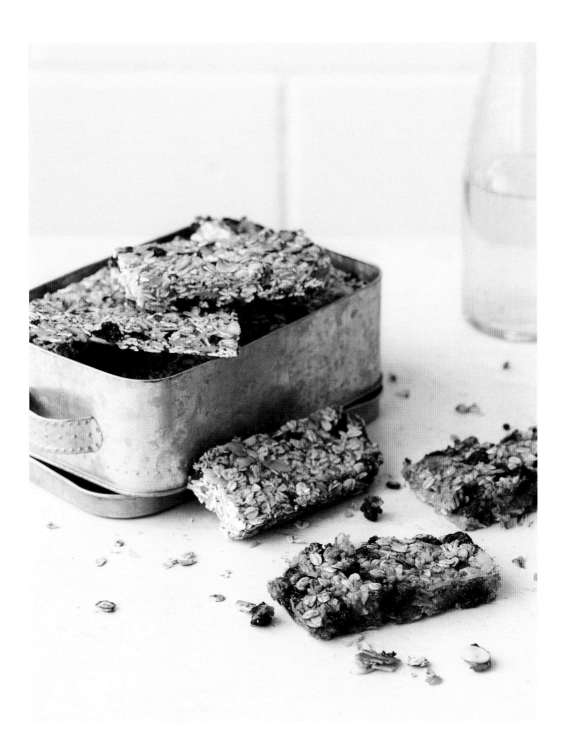

SPICED PEARS POACHED IN HONEY

Having a piece of fruit as a dessert can get boring, so here's a way to mix things up a bit with a recipe that feels much naughtier than it actually is.

Serves 4

900ml water
120ml clear honey
10cm piece fresh ginger, peeled and sliced
½ teaspoon whole cloves
1 star anise pod, broken in half
1 cinnamon stick, broken in half
4 ripe pears, peeled

Bring the water and honey gently to the boil in a large pan on the hob over a low-to-medium heat, stirring to dissolve the honey, then reduce to a simmer. Add the ginger slices, cloves, star anise and cinnamon and leave to gently cook for 10 minutes.

While the poaching liquid is simmering, take the pears and cut lengthways, leaving the stems in place. Scoop out the lower portion of the core, with the seeds. Place the pears into the liquid and turn the heat down to its lowest setting. Poach the pears for 25 minutes.

Once cooked, put the pears and poaching liquid into an airtight container and allow to cool.

Lisa's tip: Once cooled, store the poached pears in the fridge. They are equally delicious served hot or cold.

Per serving 138cals | 0g protein | 0g fat (0g saturates) | 33g carbs (33g total sugars) | 3g fibre

FRUITY FLAPJACKS

People think flapjacks are loaded with rubbish, and sadly some of the shop-bought ones are. But these are all natural, and are great as an every-now-and-again, after-dinner treat. But I do mean every now and again.

Makes 12 flapjacks

2 ripe bananas, mashed
160g porridge oats
140ml semi-skimmed milk
100g mixed nuts, chopped
50g raisins
50g coconut flakes
100g frozen berries
1 tablespoon clear honey

Preheat the oven to 160°C/Fan 140°C/Gas 3.

In a large bowl mix all of the ingredients together until well combined. Leave to stand for 10 minutes so the milk can be absorbed a little.

Line a 25cm x 30cm rectangular cake tin with greaseproof paper and pour the mixture into the tin. Smooth it out so the mixture is as flat and even as possible. Bake in the oven for 40 minutes, or until the flapjack mixture is golden brown.

Remove from the oven and place on a cooling rack. Divide into 12 slices, and serve at room temperature.

Per serving 172cals | 4g protein | 8g fat (3g saturates) | 19g carbs (9g total sugars) | 2g fibre

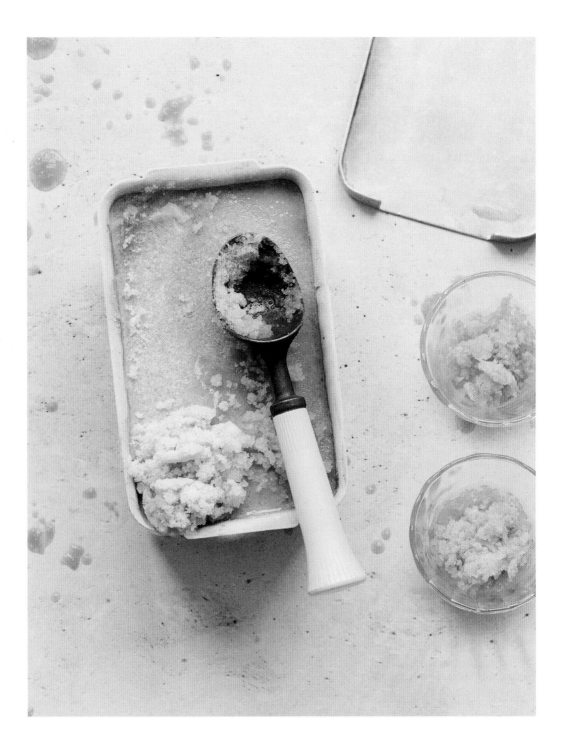

MELON SORBET

This is an incredibly simple sorbet recipe. It will take you a matter of minutes to make, and it's the perfect after-dinner palate cleanser.

Serves 6

2 fresh cantaloupe
melons, cubed

1 tablespoon lemon juice,
freshly squeezed

2 tablespoons clear honey

2 tablespoons water (and
more as needed)

½ egg white (optional)

Place the melon into a food processor along with the lemon juice, honey and water. Blitz for 3 minutes until broken down and smooth. Transfer to a freezable container and put into the freezer overnight.

The next day, return the sorbet to the food processor and blitz again to break down the ice crystals. If you like, you can add half an egg white as you blitz the sorbet for a smoother texture.

Return to the container and refreeze for a few hours.

Lisa's tip: This delicious dessert can be stored in the freezer for three to four weeks.

Per serving 54cals | 1g protein | 0g fat (0g saturates) | 10g carbs (10g total sugars) | 3g fibre

COFFEE AND WALNUT CAKE

This is strictly for the end of your diet! I've kept it as healthy as a coffee and walnut cake can be, and when you reach your goal weight you'll definitely deserve a slice. However, your slice should never be bigger than the space between the bottom of your baby finger and your knuckle. We've heard of finger sandwiches, but from now on you'll be having finger cakes, too.

Serves 12

For the cake:

1 teaspoon bicarbonate of soda
175g self-raising flour
175g light muscovado sugar
50ml vegetable oil
1 teaspoon vanilla extract
60g chopped walnuts
2 tablespoons instant coffee, dissolved in 4 tablespoons hot water
6 tablespoons low-fat yoghurt
2 egg whites

For the icing:

2 teaspoons instant coffee, dissolved in 2 tablespoons hot water
100g icing sugar, sieved
20g chopped walnuts

Preheat the oven to 180°C/Fan 160°C/Gas 4. Line a 18cm square cake tin with greaseproof paper and set to one side.

Sift the bicarbonate of soda and flour into a large bowl and then stir in the sugar, followed by the vegetable oil, vanilla essence, walnuts, coffee mixture and yoghurt.

Beat the egg whites to soft peaks in another bowl and fold them carefully into the cake mixture. Once combined, spoon the cake mixture into the lined cake tin, levelling the surface with a wooden spoon.

Place in the oven and bake for around 30–35 minutes, or until you can insert a skewer into the centre of the cake and it comes out clean.

Remove the cake from the oven and place on a cooling rack. Ensure that you remove the greaseproof paper while the cake is still warm, otherwise it will stick.

To make the icing, mix the coffee and water mixture with the sieved icing sugar in a bowl until smooth. Add drops of water, if you need to, in order to get the right spreadable consistency. Spread the coffee icing evenly over the top of the cooled cake (if it's not completely cool, the icing could slide off) and decorate with the remaining chopped walnuts.

As soon as the icing has set, you can cut the cake into 12 delicious slices!

Per serving 234cals | 4g protein | 8g fat (1g saturates) | 36g carbs (24g total sugars) | 1g fibre

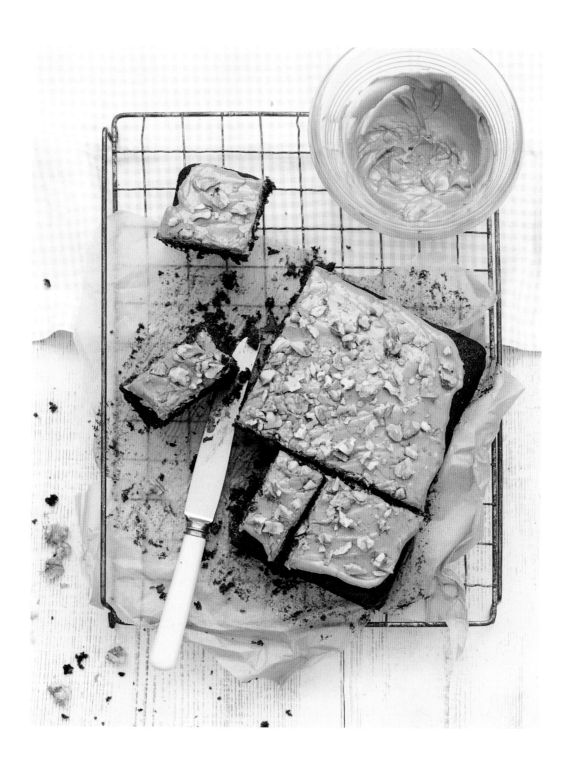

INDEX

USEFUL RESOURCES

NHS CHOICES LIVE WELL – www.nhs.uk/livewell – has information on healthy eating, weight-loss plans and support communities, as well as a calorie checker.

WEIGHT CONCERN – www.weightconcern.org.uk – provides excellent information on obesity issues, including a section on children's health and a BMI calculator.

WEIGHT LOSS RESOURCES – www.weightlossresources.co.uk – provides excellent information on weight loss, fitness and healthy eating as well as a comprehensive calorie database and a personalized weight-loss programme.

DIABETES UK – www.diabetes.org.uk – is the leading charity for people with diabetes, providing authoritative information on living with diabetes, including sections for children, teenagers and young adults.

BEAT (BEAT EATING DISORDERS) – www.b-eat.co.uk – provides helplines, online support and a network of UK-wide self-help groups, as well as downloadable information sheets and booklets.

To find a registered nutritionist visit www.associationfornutrition.org

ACKNOWLEDGEMENTS

Thank you to Jordan Paramor for taking every single good bit of me and turning it into the best dish ever. Thanks for getting me. You have been wonderful. #FRIENDFORLIFE

Thank you to Ione Walder for thinking my story was one that was worth telling, and to Amy and everyone else at Michael Joseph who worked so hard on the book.

And a big thank you to the other people who also made this book happen, including my manager, Phil Dale. The dream team strikes again. We're still in the premiership! And to Shirley Patton from ITV: your support has meant so much.

Masses of appreciation to Sarah Murch from Blakeway TV, who allowed me to make *Lisa Riley's Baggy Body Club*, so that I was able to help people who are on a similar journey to me. I'll always be grateful I kissed the Blarney Stone!

Thank you to my incredible surgeon, Rob Winterton, Bev and all the staff at Spire Hospital, Manchester. Stacey, I'll never ever forget what you did for me.

To Yolanda and Nana: thank you for making me realize that cooking is more than just confidence. It's self-belief, and you both gave me that.

I have so many other people I'd like to thank, but really this book is also for everyone who believed in me. I could list hundreds, but you all know who you are. You've all changed my life in some small way and that means everything to me.

Loads of love,
Lisa xxx